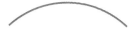

WHY
TONGUE-TIE
MATTERS

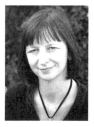

About the author

Sarah Oakley has been in nursing for over 30 years, qualifying as a Registered General Nurse in 1991 and as a Health Visitor in 2003. After qualifying in 2009 as an International Board Certified Lactation Consultant she set up in private practice offering specialist infant feeding support. In 2011 Sarah trained to perform tongue-tie division in babies with feeding issues and has built up a very busy infant feeding support practice since seeing 600-700 families per year in Cambridgeshire, Norfolk and Suffolk. Sarah also provides training in tongue-tie and infant feeding to breastfeeding supporters and healthcare professionals and has worked with several NHS Trusts providing training on tongue-tie identification and management. She has also spoken at national and international conferences. She is a founder member and former Chair of the Association of Tongue-tie Practitioners in the UK.

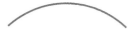

WHY
TONGUE-TIE
MATTERS

Sarah Oakley

pinter & martin

Why Tongue-tie Matters (Pinter & Martin Why It Matters 22)

First published by Pinter & Martin Ltd 2021

ISBN 978-1-78066-645-7

Also available as an ebook

Pinter & Martin Why It Matters ISSN 2056-8657

Series editor: Susan Last
Index: Helen Bilton
Cover Design: Blok Graphic, London
Cover Illustration: Lucy Davey
Illustrations page 18: Salma Price-Nell at thesalsacreative.com

British Library Cataloguing-in-Publication Data
A catalogue record for this book is available from the British Library.

Set in Minion

Printed and bound in the EU by Hussar

This book has been printed on paper that is sourced and harvested from sustainable forests and is FSC accredited.

Pinter & Martin Ltd
6 Effra Parade
London SW2 1PS

pinterandmartin.com

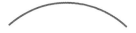

Contents

Introduction   7

1 What is a tongue-tie?   15
2 The impact of tongue-tie on infant feeding   27
3 Assessment and diagnosis of tongue-tie   55
4 Treatment of tongue-tie   70
5 Strategies to help a tongue-tied baby feed
   before and after division   105
6 Myths and controversies   127
7 When treatment doesn't improve things   138

Appendix   144
Acknowledgements   147
References   148
Index   154

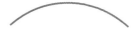

Introduction

I have found writing this introduction a struggle. As someone who has studied the anatomy and physiology of infant feeding, read the research, sees daily the impact tongue-tie has on infant feeding (and maternal mental health) and witnesses how a simple procedure to divide the tongue-tie can transform the situation, I find it hard to understand why this issue still attracts so much controversy.

'Why isn't tongue-tie checked for at birth?' I provide daily clinics assessing and treating babies for tongue-tie, run a weekly breastfeeding support group and admin a tongue-tie support group on Facebook, so I get a lot of practice answering this question. But somehow, the explanations I give seem inadequate and don't always make a lot of sense to parents.

The simple answer is that assessment for tongue-tie is not part of the Newborn and Infant Physical Examination (NIPE), which is the top-to-toe examination performed within 6–72 hours of birth by a paediatrician, neonatal nurse or midwife. This examination screens for abnormalities of the eyes, hips, heart and testes, but is a full examination of the baby, including visual inspection of the palate, gums and tongue and assessment of the sucking reflex. However, a visual inspection of the tongue tells us nothing about tongue function or whether there is a tongue-tie. Furthermore, the training for staff who perform this examination does not include tongue-tie assessment.

So why isn't tongue-tie included in the NIPE, when every other aspect of a baby's health and wellbeing is so closely examined, monitored and measured?

Assessing for tongue-tie is not something that can be incorporated into the top-to-toe check when the expectation is that the whole process will take no more than about 30 minutes. To identify a tongue-tie not only does the function and appearance of the tongue need to be assessed, but also a feed needs to be observed and a detailed feeding history taken. Often getting a true picture of any issues involves a period of several feeds, perhaps over several days or even weeks. Assessment for tongue-tie is a dynamic process, as the effects of a tongue-tie are not always immediately evident but evolve over time. Some of the more restrictive tongue-ties will very clearly need dividing early on, but this is not always the case with every tongue-tie. In a sample of 201 babies born with tongue-tie in Southampton, only 88 experienced difficulties with breast or bottle-feeding and required division (Hogan, Westcott, & Griffiths, 2005). This highlights the importance of a feeding assessment.

The next question that often comes from parents is, 'Why did no one check for tongue-tie when I told them about all the feeding difficulties I was having?' This is tougher to answer, because it is not at all unreasonable to expect that your midwife, health visitor, GP, or indeed the infant feeding specialist at the hospital where your baby was born, or those staffing clinics and groups out in the community, should be competent in recognising when tongue-tie may be an issue and assessing for it. However, this is not the case.

I put out a short two-question survey on my Facebook page in December 2019 asking parents who had identified their baby's tongue-tie. I closed the survey at 100 responses. Only a third of the babies in my survey were diagnosed by healthcare professionals, with 18% being diagnosed by private IBCLCs, and 16% being identified in breastfeeding groups run by volunteers. Obviously this is a somewhat skewed sample, as many of my page followers will have used my private lactation consultant and tongue-tie service. However, it demonstrates that a significant number of parents are having to look beyond the skills of healthcare professionals when it comes to tongue-tie. Almost a third of parents (27%) reported that they had spotted the tongue-tie themselves!

The National Institute for Health and Care Excellence (NICE) issued guidance on Maternal and Child Nutrition in 2008 and this was subsequently updated (NICE, 2014). Recommendations 7–12 relate to breastfeeding. They talk about a multifaceted approach across different settings, with joint working between paid professionals and volunteers, to increase breastfeeding rates. They also identify the importance of training for healthcare professionals and peer supporters and the implementation of structured programmes such as the UNICEF Baby Friendly Initiative as the minimum standard. There is a whole recommendation devoted to the expressing and storage of breastmilk. But there are no specific recommendations relating to tongue-tie, and the only reference to it is a link to the NICE Guidance *Division of Ankyloglossia (tongue-tie) for breastfeeding* (NICE, 2005) in the 'Related NICE Guidance' section. For an issue that is thought to affect around one in ten babies (Hogan, Westcott, & Griffiths, 2005) and can seriously jeopardise breastfeeding and negatively impact bottle-feeding, you may find this surprising.

So why is the issue being overlooked? Providing skilled infant feeding support to all families from birth and throughout the first year of life, so problems related to tongue-tie can be identified and managed appropriately and in a timely way, requires a considerable amount of investment in staff, training and resources. Herein lies part of the problem. Despite the acknowledgement of the importance of breastfeeding within official guidance both nationally and internationally (WHO, 2003) infant feeding is an area of healthcare that has always suffered from underinvestment. It is not seen as a priority. To some extent the emergence of the highly skilled and dedicated voluntary breastfeeding sector since the 1950s, first with La Leche League and then the Association of Breastfeeding Mothers and more recently Breastfeeding Network, has let the policymakers and purse-string holders off the hook.

Infant feeding education does not feature highly in the training of doctors, midwives and health visitors. Medical students get just seven hours on child nutrition and the emphasis is on medicalised feeding interventions such as nasogastric and gastrostomy feeding.

As a student health visitor back in 2002/3 I got just three hours on breastfeeding, and this was organised by our tutor as an 'extra' session. No specific mention is made of infant feeding in the *Standards of Proficiency for Specialist Community Public Health Nurses (Health Visitors)* (NMC, 2004). The initiation and continuation of breastfeeding is one of the Essential Skills Clusters within the *Standards for Pre-registration Midwifery Education* (NMC, 2009). However, the training offered to midwives and some health visitors as part of the pre-registration courses, or subsequently once qualified, is the UNICEF Baby Friendly Breastfeeding Management Course (15 hours), which focuses on supporting the healthy full-term baby to breastfeed and does not address more complex situations, including tongue-tie, in depth. This does not compare well with the training and experience of International Board Certified Lactation Consultants (IBCLCs), for example, who have a minimum of 90 hours of taught lactation education, 1,000 hours of breastfeeding counselling experience and sit a four-hour exam (IBLCE, 2019).

There are relatively few IBCLCs employed in the NHS, so access to this level of support is limited and many parents pay for it privately. Where IBCLCs are employed in NHS settings they are usually also qualified midwives or health visitors and as such have many other pressures on their time.

Alison Hazelbaker, an American IBCLC, writes in her book (Hazelbaker, 2010) about a nurse/lactation consultant colleague's experience:

> *Last year I saw the worst tongue-tied baby I have ever seen… I went to the M.D. who was caring for the baby… and asked him if he would take a look and determine if the baby needed an ENT* [Ear, nose and throat] *consult. He went ballistic. He said that the tongue has nothing at all to do with breastfeeding… He then went to my manager and wanted me fired or reprimanded.*

After discussing this with my NHS colleagues it seems this experience is not unique to the USA. One midwife colleague told me, 'I got a written warning for identifying issues which may be affecting latch! Needless to say, I ultimately lost my job over this embargo on diagnosing tongue-ties'. Another colleague told me that after asking for more hours to run extra tongue-tie clinics she was told to only do the 'serious' ones. What was she to tell the parents of the babies with 'less serious' tongue-ties who were struggling with feeding? Any tongue-tie that is impacting feeding is significant, so how can some be disregarded?

Why would midwives, health visitors, IBCLCs be put under this pressure to keep quiet when they suspect or notice a tongue-tie? After all, it would be a disciplinary matter if healthcare professionals overlooked, failed to tell parents or failed to investigate when a baby had symptoms of a heart murmur, a dislocated hip, or an undescended testicle.

Historically there has been scepticism among the medical profession when it comes to tongue-tie. Nils Rosen von Rosenstein, Swedish Royal Physician, wrote in 1776: 'When children do not work well our old women say that they are tongue-tied and pretend that the bridle ought to be snipped with a pair of scissors. I have never as yet seen any child's tongue tied…' (cited by Callum, 1959). This comment demonstrates not only a scepticism about the existence of tongue-tie, but also a lack of trust and respect for the opinions and experiences of women.

Some of the current barriers to having tongue-tie acknowledged as a feeding issue are the result of the unregulated promotion of formula-feeding which went on from the 1950s until the 1980s, and which led to a drop in breastfeeding rates and a devaluing of breastfeeding. Along with this came the demise of tongue-tie division in infants struggling to feed as the perception was that tongue-tie didn't impact bottle-feeding (although it can and does). Prior to this, tongue-tie division to resolve breastfeeding issues seems to have been carried out routinely and had been since at least the eighteenth century and probably before that. Callum (1959) in his article on tongue-tie published in the *British Medical Journal* cites a reference to tongue-tie in infants from 1697. He goes on to cite an essay by Liverpool surgeon William Moss from 1794, who wrote:

A child's being tongue tied will impede and hinder his sucking freely. When that happens he may be observed to lose his hold very often, and when he draws the breast he frequently makes a chucking noise. Upon this occasion the mouth must be examined and the tongue set at liberty by cutting a ligament or string which will be found to confine the tongue down to the lower part of the mouth and which is done by the surgeon with little or no pain to the child who will commonly take the breast immediately after the operation without any further inconvenience to him and there never is any danger to be apprehended from bleeding or any other consequence of the operation. One out of three or four children are tongue-tied more or less.

In recent years the development of a Global Strategy on Infant and Young Child Nutrition by the World Health Organisation (WHO, 2003), and the introduction of the UNICEF Baby Friendly Initiative (UNICEF BFI, 1992), along with the advocacy of the voluntary breastfeeding sector and the development of the role of the IBCLC has revived our knowledge of breastfeeding. Inevitably this led to a re-examination of the issue of tongue-tie, with some surgeons performing the procedure again, including Mervyn Griffiths in Southampton (who went on to publish research on the efficacy of division which informed the 2005 NICE Guidance).

However, some medical professionals have remained resistant to the idea that tongue-tie impacts infant feeding and should be treated. Indeed, when Mervyn Griffiths first put forward his research for publication in a medical journal, he was reported by that journal to his medical director for performing unethical procedures. My own GP threatened to report me for carrying out division because as a self-employed nurse he believed I was not allowed to and the paediatricians at the local hospital had told him it was an unnecessary procedure. A survey carried out in 2000 in the USA found

13

that 90% of paediatricians believed tongue-tie rarely or never causes feeding difficulties (A Messner & Lalakea, 2000).

This potted history is intended to show why parents seeking solutions to infant feeding issues, particularly when tongue-tie is involved, may face difficulties. The rest of the book aims to provide information and support that may help to improve this situation.

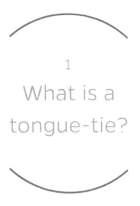

1

What is a tongue-tie?

As you read through this book you will come to realise that everything about tongue-tie is controversial. This even applies to how we define a tongue-tie.

For many years we all believed that the lingual frenulum (the stringy bit that stretches from the under surface of our tongue to the floor of the mouth) was composed of a discreet strand or band of mucous membrane. A tongue-tie (or restricted lingual frenulum) was defined in terms of this strand or band of mucous membrane being abnormally short or tight, or attached close to the tip of the tongue and thereby limiting tongue movement.

Jack Newman, a Canadian paediatrician who specialises in breastfeeding wrote in 2000:

Under the tongue we all have a whitish vertical strip of tissue called the frenulum, which attaches to the floor of our mouth at one end and to the tongue at the other. When the frenulum is tight, it can prevent the baby from getting his tongue well forward to cup under the breast and extract the milk.

UNICEF provides this description on the Babyfriendly website www.unicef.org.uk/babyfriendly/support-for-parents/tongue-tie (accessed 30/3/2020):

Many babies have a piece of membrane under their tongue (the frenulum), which does not usually cause problems. Tongue-tie (ankyloglossia) occurs when the frenulum is abnormally short, stopping the tip of the tongue from protruding beyond the lower gum. This may cause problems with feeding as a result of the inability to move the tongue in a normal way and therefore attach and suck effectively. The frenulum may reach the tip of the tongue and be easily seen and may be either thin and stretchy or thicker/tighter. A posterior frenulum, which is at the back of the tongue, can be less easy to see and in some cases may only be felt.

However, in recent years we have had to start rethinking this in light of three new research papers which looked at the anatomy of the lingual frenulum. The first was published in 2013 in Brazil (Martinelli et al, 2013) where assessing newborns for tongue-tie is a statutory requirement. After assessing a sample of 50 school-age children, the study authors identified eight as having altered lingual frenula using a tool developed by Irene Marcheson, a speech and language pathologist. These children underwent surgery to remove the lingual frenulum and the frenula tissue was examined under a microscope. They found that the lingual frenulum is made up of the same tissue as the rest of the oral mucosa. However, the restricted lingual frenula (those restricting function of the tongue) had significant bundles of muscle fibres scattered on the fold of the mucosa with a high frequency of collagen type one fibres. Collagen type one is not stretchy, so the frenulum was causing restriction in tongue function. Those frenula that were identified as posterior (attached towards the back of the underside of the tongue and not so easy to see) and short also contained more muscle fibres. The anterior frenula (those attached close to the tongue-tie and visibly obvious), even if they were short, were similar in structure to oral mucosa.

So, from this study we learnt that not all lingual frenula are the same in terms of their structure and this has implications for division and healing. While mucous membrane is unlikely to form scar tissue, as Alison Hazelbaker describes in her book (2010), structures containing collagen and muscle fibres may be more likely to. This shone light on the fact that thicker, more posterior tongue-ties seem, anecdotally, more prone to recurrence, which is something we will explore later in this book. It also means that the idea, often perpetuated by GPs and paediatricians, that the tongue-tie will stretch on its own, is less likely.

In 2019 two further studies were published by a team led by ENT Surgeon Nikki Mills in New Zealand. These examined the in situ lingual frenulum in both babies and adults. The researchers describe the lingual frenulum as a dynamic structure, formed by a midline fold in a layer of fascia that inserts around the inner arc of the lower jaw, forming a skirt like structure across the floor of mouth. You can see this 'skirt' fanning out across the floor of your own mouth if you lift your tongue and look in a mirror. This fascia is immediately below the oral mucosal layer and beneath this there are muscle fibres. The graphics overleaf demonstrate the layered structure of the lingual frenulum, as described by Nikki Mills and her team (2019), and how lingual frenula can vary in structure.

This helps to explains why the wounds we achieve with division can vary in appearance, size and depth and why some wounds bleed more than others and why some form

Thin lingual frenulum composed predominantly of mucous membrane

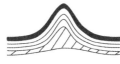
mucous membrane
fascia
muscle

Thicker lingual frenulum with the layer of fascia being drawn up into the fold of mucous membrane

Thick lingual frenulum with the layers of fascia and muscle being drawn up into the fold of mucous membrane

Graphic demonstrating the layered nature of the lingual frenulum as highlighted in the studies by Mills et al (2019)

more scarring than others and may be more likely to reoccur. One of the skills of a practitioner is to know just how much traction to apply when lifting the tongue so as not to pull up the muscle tissue, which is certainly not always easy when you are working in such a tiny mouth.

So how do we differentiate between a normal lingual frenulum and a tongue-tie (restricted lingual frenulum)? This is a source of ongoing debate and research. Lingual frenula differ in appearance as the images opposite show.

Generally lingual frenula that are attached posteriorly (towards the base of the tongue), are thin, long (1.5cm or more) and elastic, are considered normal anatomy based on Alison Hazelbaker's Assessment Tool for Lingual Frenulum Function (2017), which can be found here: www.alisonhazelbaker.com/shop/hatlff-hazelbaker-assessment-tool-for-lingual-frenulum-

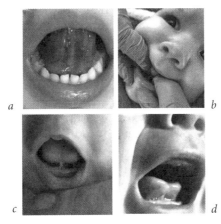

A is a normal lingual frenulum, B and C are both restricted lingual frenula attached close to the tip of the tongue. D is a lingual frenulum which is attached midway along the under surface of the tongue.

function. However, a lingual frenulum attached close to the tongue tip may not always cause significant problems with feeding, as noted in a randomised control trial published by Monica Hogan, Carolyn Westcott and Mervyn Griffith (2005) and of course a visible lingual frenulum is normal anatomy so we need to look at function.

Function is assessed using various tools which we will explore later. A study looking at the Hazelbaker tool concluded that tongue extension, lateralisation and elevation are reliable indicators of the severity of a tongue-tie. Indeed, all the published tools require an assessment of the baby's ability to lift the tongue and extend the tongue. Tongue lift seems to be the most crucial indicator. It is usually assessed when a baby is crying. The consensus is that the tongue tip needs to be able to lift to mid-mouth or higher with the mouth wide open. Some babies with tongue-tie will struggle to open their mouths wide due to the tension created by the restricted lingual frenulum. They have what we call the characteristic 'letter box' mouth when crying. Babies with tongue-tie will often not be able to lift their tongues off the floor of the mouth at all. Some will be able to lift the side edges but not the tip, so the tongue will from a 'V' shape. Others will curl up the edges but not lift the posterior part of the tongue, so the tongue forms a bowl shape. The ability of the baby to lift the tongue up and down during feeding is key to creating the necessary vacuum to remove milk from the breast (Geddes et al, 2008). So poor elevation impacts efficiency, which can lead to poor weight gain and a drop in milk supply if a baby is breastfed.

The inability of a baby to extend their tongue beyond the bottom lip is also hugely significant in cases of breastfeeding difficulty. If a baby cannot extend their tongue adequately, they struggle to latch to the breast and sustain the latch at the breast and will compress the nipple, causing pain and damage. Nipple pain is by far the most common consequence of a tongue-tie. However, I have seen babies where a restriction in tongue extension has been related to strain within the neck which has developed during the birth. In these babies the lingual frenulum often looks normal and tongue elevation is good.

Research using ultrasound conducted in Brazil emphasises the role of the tongue in breastfeeding (Elad et al 2014):

We have shown, for the first time to our knowledge, that latch-on to draw the nipple–areola complex into the infant mouth, as well as milk extraction during breast-feeding, require development of time-varying sub atmospheric pressures within the infant's oral cavity. Analysis of the US movies clearly demonstrated that tongue motility during breast-feeding was fairly periodic. The anterior tongue, which is wedged between the nipple–areola complex and the lower lips, moves as a rigid body with the cycling motion of the mandible, while the posterior section of the tongue undulates in a pattern similar to a propagating peristaltic wave, which is essential for swallowing.

Simply put, babies need to first be able to open their mouths wide to latch to the breast, while simultaneously bringing their tongue down and forward over the bottom lip, creating a groove to scoop up the breast. The nipple and areola are then drawn in by negative pressure. Negative pressure is generated when the anterior (front) part of the tongue moves up and down, compressing the nipple against the hard palate, and the posterior (rear) part of the tongue drops, creating a peristaltic (wave-like) motion. This movement of the tongue is driven by the oscillation of the lower jaw and the resulting negative pressure is crucial as it is responsible for removing milk from the breast.

Causes of tongue-tie

Lingual frenula had been thought to result from incomplete tissue degeneration (apoptosis) during the first nine weeks of pregnancy as the embryo forms, and this would explain the wide variations in the appearance of lingual frenula. However, the New Zealand papers (Mills, et al, 2019) on lingual frenulum anatomy call this into question and so a tongue-tie may just be a normal variant. Alison Hazelbaker (2010) cites several papers which support the idea that tongue-ties run in families and I see this myself in practice. So, both genetic and environmental factors are thought to be at play.

Parents will often come across information suggesting a link between folic acid supplementation prior to conception and in pregnancy with tongue-tie, and this theory has been linked to a mutation of the MTHFR gene. This gene mutation is common, affecting 30–40% of the American population according to information on the US National Library of Medicine website. This gene provides instructions for an enzyme involved in the conversion of folate. It is thought that the mutation causes issues with the metabolism of folic acid, leading to a deficiency in folate, and that this can cause tongue-tie. However, there is no evidence at the time of writing to back up this idea, although it is an area of ongoing research. Two papers have been published. One looked at maternal folic acid consumption and found no link with oral findings, including tongue-tie, in newborns (Perez-Aguire et al, 2018). The other looked at maternal intake of folic acid before conception and found that those mothers with a tongue-tied baby reported taking folic acid on a 'regular' basis more frequently than the mothers in the control group (Amitai et al, 2019). But the numbers in both studies were small, so no conclusions can be drawn, and in view of the well-established link between neural tube defects (spina bifida) and folic acid deficiency, guidelines on supplementation both before conception and in pregnancy should be adhered to. Anecdotally, one of the most restrictive tongue-ties I have ever seen was in a baby whose mum told me she had never taken folic acid! Furthermore, the apparent rise in the number of tongue-ties has occurred alongside the introduction and growing awareness of the need for folic acid supplements in the preconception and early pregnancy period, so what may seem like an association may just be coincidence.

Another less well-known theory explored by dentist Dr Steven Lin in his article 'Is tongue-tie genetic? Here is the truth' is that tongue-tie may be linked to a deficiency in vitamin A. Vitamin A plays a role in facial development and activates genes involved in apoptosis and cell death so this theory is plausible, but not of course if tongue-ties are just a normal variant. Regardless, we need to be cautious about vitamin A supplementation because Dr Lin also cites an association between excess vitamin A and cleft defects.

How common is tongue-tie?

Parents often ask, 'How common is tongue-tie?' Some parents report that neither they nor their families or friends have ever heard of tongue-tie. Others tell me that within their circle of friends almost everyone has had a baby with a tongue-tie. If you are not aware, as a professional, of tongue-tie as a potential cause of feeding difficulties, you won't look for it and it will go unnoticed. This was the case for a long period between the 1950s and the early 2000s.

Prior to the 1950s, before formula feeding was aggressively marketed and promoted, tongue-tie was recognised as a feeding issue and was treated as discussed in the Introduction. Cullum, in his article on tongue-tie in infancy, published in the *British Medical Journal* in 1959, cites rates of one in four children being affected. Indeed, some of my colleagues in the USA would concur with this estimate based on what they are seeing today.

However, it is incredibly difficult to get accurate figures on incidence. It really depends on which study you look at. Ingram et al (2015) quote an incidence range of 3–16%. Why such variation? Given that the cause of tongue-tie is thought to be rooted in genetics it is not surprising that incidence will vary in different populations.

Other factors which contribute to the wide variation include a lack of consensus on how best to assess and diagnose a tongue-tie. What constitutes a normal lingual frenulum and an abnormal (or restricted) lingual frenulum is open to interpretation and the criteria used to assess function vary across the published tools and in the practice of individual professionals. How much tongue extension or tongue elevation is adequate is not easy to define, because breastfeeding involves the mother and not just the baby. Her anatomy will also have an influence over how easily her baby can latch and feed at the breast. For example, a baby with a mild restriction in tongue extension may be able to latch easily and comfortably if the nipple is prominent and elastic. That same baby may not be able to latch at all if the nipple is very flat or inverted. We see this demonstrated in practice when a baby latches well to one breast but not the other due to the variation in nipple anatomy. Other aspects of the baby's oral anatomy may also have an influence on the degree of breastfeeding difficulty. A baby with a recessed lower jaw may struggle more to latch with a mild restriction in tongue extension as the lower jaw being set further back means the tongue has further to travel when coming down and forward to latch.

There is no clear consensus and standardised diagnostic criteria for tongue-tie so studies looking at incidence will draw different conclusions depending on the diagnostic criteria or assessment tool they have chosen to use. Earlier studies tended to look only at 'anterior' type tongue-ties (those that are attached close to the tongue tip and are visually obvious). The concept of 'posterior', or 'sub-mucosal' tongue-tie (where the frenulum is attached further back at the base of the tongue and is not visually obvious) was not put forward until 2004 when it was first defined by Betty Coryllos and Catherine Watson Genna. So, these would not have been identified within those studies but may have been included in later ones.

A study done in the UK in 2002 (Hogan et al, 2005) found an incidence of 10.8%, but interestingly only around half of these babies (43%) with a tongue-tie were reported to need a division. In a study of 200 babies in Brazil (Haham, 2014) the rate of division was 3.5% and David Todd and Monica Hogan (2015) quote a rate of 4.7–5.0% in their audit of practice at a hospital in Canberra, Australia. So, working on the basis that around one in 20 babies will need a division would seem reasonable based on these studies. But a more recent study conducted in 2018 in Spain (Maya-Enero et al, 2020) with a sample of 1,392 newborns, used the Hazelbaker tool (which we will look at later) to assess those babies where the mother had nipple pain or bruising, or the baby had difficulty latching. This study identified 645 babies as having a tongue-tie, with 453 being symptomatic (32.5%). This is considerably higher (one in three) than the one in 20 indicated from other studies. The explosion in numbers of divisions being reported, whether justified or not, has led to concerns being raised about over treatment, particularly in the USA and Australia.

When I first started dividing tongue-ties in 2011, I rarely had a baby attend who did not have an obvious, significant tongue-tie. Now at least a fifth of the babies that come to me for division either do not have a tongue-tie or have a very mild restriction with minor feeding difficulties which can be resolved with conservative strategies. I have had a case where a surgeon told a mother he could not find a frenulum to cut but would obtain a Brodie director (a grooved spade-shaped instrument used to lift the tongue) to see if he could isolate a frenulum that way. The baby had multiple other structural issues going on which would have been impacting feeding. But these were all overlooked in pursuit of a tongue-tie. I have also had a case where the baby's weight loss was attributed to a posterior tongue-tie. However, on full assessment I was able to identify mammary hypoplasia (a lack of breast tissue development at puberty which can cause low milk supply in varying degrees) as the cause of the weight loss. The mother had had breast implants as she simply never developed any breasts, and she never produced more than a few drops of milk. Her baby did have a posterior tongue-tie with a mild restriction, but dividing it was not going to lead to her being able to breastfeed her baby. This was utterly heart-breaking for her and a difficult discussion for us both. But she said it also gave her some peace as she had a similar experience with her first baby, who ended up formula-fed due to early weight loss, and she had never understood why. Anyone referring babies for division or performing tongue-tie division needs expertise in infant feeding and tongue-tie assessment, or should be working alongside someone who has.

These cases demonstrate how the tongue-tie issue can dominate our thought processes and I have no doubt that some unnecessary procedures are being carried out. As a private practitioner I have been accused of this. Anyone providing private healthcare is always regarded with suspicion in the UK and can expect their motives to be questioned. However, tongue-tie clinics can be a useful income generator for NHS hospitals too, so commercial influence may be present whatever the setting.

Notwithstanding this, I still see a significant number of older babies with long histories of feeding difficulties where a tongue-tie has been repeatedly missed. I also see cases in younger babies where it has only been picked up because of the tenacity and persistence of parents who have done their own research and sought help from multiple sources. These experiences can be harrowing for parents and should be deeply concerning to professionals. This is why tongue-tie matters. We owe it to babies and parents to get it right. We cannot encourage parents to breastfeed their babies exclusively for six months and to continue into toddlerhood as per the WHO Recommendation on Infant Feeding (2001) and then overlook a relatively common anatomical issue which may make exclusive, full-term breastfeeding impossible. We have a lot more to learn, and as you continue to read through this book you will see there are still unanswered questions and uncertainties in this field. Like many issues that affect predominantly women and babies, tongue-tie is under-researched and misunderstood, even though we know tongue-ties have been affecting babies for centuries and probably for much longer.

2

The impact of tongue-tie on infant feeding

As discussed in the last chapter babies need to be able to open their mouths wide to latch to the breast, while simultaneously bringing their tongue down and forward over the bottom lip, creating a groove to scoop up the breast. The nipple and areola are then drawn in by negative pressure. Negative pressure is generated when the anterior (front) part of the tongue moves up and down, compressing the nipple against the hard palate, and the posterior (rear) part of the tongue drops, creating a peristaltic (wave-like) motion. This movement of the tongue is driven by the oscillation of the lower jaw and the resulting negative pressure is crucial as it is responsible for removing milk from the breast.

The tongue tip needs to be able to extend beyond the lip to locate the breast and form a groove for the baby to scoop up the breast and latch on easily. The baby then needs to maintain the tongue tip over the lower gum to cushion the nipple. The ability to keep the tongue forwards over the gum also helps the baby to sustain a secure latch at the breast, along with cupping of the tongue. Cupping of the tongue refers to the baby in effect 'hugging' the breast tissue with their tongue. The side edges of the tongue wrap round the breast tissue, so the tongue forms a 'U' shape. Not only does this 'hugging' of the breast tissue help the baby to sustain a secure latch, but it also helps the baby to create a seal at the breast, along with the lips. Difficulty in creating a seal can be seen when babies dribble milk during feeds.

Some babies will be able to extend their tongues sufficiently to latch easily. But they struggle to maintain the tongue in a forward position over the gum due to the tension created by the tongue-tie, and the tongue will snap back behind the gum. This can create a clicking sound, due to loss of contact and suction, which can be heard during feeding in some babies with tongue-ties and is sometimes the first symptom to be noted. When the tongue slips back this means the nipple is exposed to the gum surface which can be extremely painful for the mother. Furthermore, as the tongue snaps back the baby will sometimes employ compensations to stay attached to the breast, rather than allowing themselves to slip off. These compensations can include employing the muscles in the lips to maintain the seal, resulting in 'cobble stone' blisters on the lips, and clamping down with the jaw, which can cause excruciating nipple pain and damage.

An inability to lift the tongue tip up and down will impact on the ability to create the wavelike motion needed to draw the nipple deep into the mouth to the junction of the soft and hard palate. This results in a shallow latch with the nipple tip being squashed up against the hard palate (roof of the mouth) causing nipple distortion, pain, and trauma. This compression of the nipple can be further exacerbated by the baby humping, rather than dropping, the posterior (back) part of the tongue (Watson Genna, 2017). At the end of a feed the nipple may look ridged, lipstick shaped, flattened and/or white (blanched). This blanching, which results from a disruption to the blood flow to the nipple due to the compressive forces from the shallow latch, can trigger a deep burning breast pain after feeds as the blood flows back into the nipple and the nipple will throb.

The ability to lift the tongue tip and drop the back of the tongue is also crucial in creating the negative pressure (vacuum) required to remove milk effectively from the breast (Geddes et al, 2008). Babies who are not able to do this will not feed efficiently and effective breast drainage will be compromised. This can make feeding very tiring for the baby and parents often report that the baby feeds constantly without being satisfied, or feeds are short but very frequent. Feeding can be such hard work for some babies that a tremor in the tongue can be felt or seen in the jaw during feeds. The ineffective drainage of the breast can trigger engorgement, blocked ducts, mastitis, and breast abscess. All the breast abscesses I recall seeing in the last 10 years have been associated with tongue-ties. These can be difficult to treat, requiring repeated aspiration or surgical drainage and long courses of antibiotics. Healing can be prolonged and painful and not surprisingly many mothers will cease breastfeeding after such an experience.

Beth describes her experience of breast abscess here:

I found a lump in my breast about a week after a bout of mastitis. Despite feeling fine and the lump not really being painful, I was still very suspicious that it was an abscess and not 'just' a blocked duct, because it was so big and the usual blocked duct clearing methods weren't having any effect. But it was difficult to get the GPs to agree to refer me to the breast clinic for investigation. I had to be very persistent over the course of a week and even then, they still were very reluctant. I am lucky that I had the energy to fight for referral. In hospital the 5cm diameter abscess was drained under ultrasound and required several outpatient visits for repeat ultrasound and drainage over the following weeks. I am so glad I trusted my intuition and pushed hard for a diagnosis, as it would otherwise have got much worse. The worst part of the whole thing was that I was on antibiotics for weeks and weeks and they upset my newborn's tummy so she had secondary lactose intolerance diarrhoea that lasted several weeks after the antibiotics had stopped.

Inefficient feeding and ineffective breast drainage will also cause a drop in milk supply and slow weight gain. In extreme cases babies may not be able to create enough vacuum to remove the milk from the breast at all. These are the babies that lose lots of weight in the first five days of life (10% or more) and will continue to lose weight or struggle to gain any weight, even after the milk has come in. Sometimes, once the milk has come in, provided there is sufficient milk and a good flow, some babies will be able to get sufficient milk simply by sucking enough to stimulate the milk ejection reflex ('let down'). This will allow the milk to 'fire hose' into their mouths. This is a passive way of feeding, reliant on the flow of milk from the mother, rather than on active transfer of milk by the baby. It works, especially in mothers with a particularly good supply (often those that have breastfed before). However, once supply naturally down-regulates and the fast flow subsides at around 4–8 weeks, we see babies who then become increasingly frustrated and fussy at the breast and in whom weight gain begins to slow. Babies who are reliant on the flow to transfer the milk also tend to be very windy and often vomit a lot after feeds. This is because the restriction in tongue movement not only impacts the ability to create vacuum and draw milk, but also the baby's ability to regulate a fast flow. So these babies gulp at the breast and sometimes cough, choke and come off, completely overwhelmed by the flow. The taking in of air (aerophagia) during feeds, due to difficulty with flow regulation and poor seal associated with tongue-tie, is thought to contribute to wind and reflux symptoms (Siegel, 2016).

Claire describes what breastfeeding a tongue-tie baby can be like:

My little boy, Lewis, wasn't feeding well from birth. For several weeks I carried on in terrible pain (sore, cracked nipples and pain when feeding as Lewis was only sucking the very end). We had a crying baby who could not get enough milk. He was attached to me a large amount of the time, probably because he was getting tiny amounts at each feed, which would last for at least 45 minutes at a time. I would try the different positions, with Lewis crying when this was attempted as it was interrupting his feeding. Some people commented (in a negative way) that he seemed to be permanently attached to my boobs which made me feel worse, like I was doing something wrong. In desperation late one night we went to A & E as nobody seemed to be listening. He was checked and a tongue-tie was ruled out. A midwife there spent some time assessing our breastfeeding and trying to show me how to do it, we tried with a nipple shield and expressing to feed from a little cup. But I left feeling defeated and no further forwards. I tried different nipple shields which I found very awkward and inconvenient, and expressed to try bottle-feeding but I had a tiny supply as there was such minimal effective feeding. My sister in law extremely kindly expressed her breastmilk so that I could bottle-feed him as well as carrying on trying to breastfeed myself, as she a had a baby a week before me and had an abundant supply. She even offered to breastfeed Lewis herself, and although I was grateful, I couldn't accept this help. I felt awful that I was unable to adequately feed my baby myself and was often in tears and had little sleep due to such constant feeding throughout the day and night. I dreaded breastfeeding because of how it made me feel both physically and mentally. And I was so worried because he was barely gaining any weight, having a low birth weight to begin with.

Bottle-fed babies

Babies who are bottle fed can often feed well despite having a tongue-tie, as they do not need such a wide range of tongue movement as a breastfed baby. A study by Catherine Watson Genna et al (2021) which utilised ultrasound to image the kinematics in both breastfeeding and bottle-feeding demonstrated that the peristaltic motion of the posterior tongue seen in breastfeeding is absent in bottle-feeding. Of course a bottle doesn't complain of pain if the teat is being rubbed by baby's gum or crushed between baby's jaws either! However, bottle-fed babies with tongue-ties can still have issues with creating a seal, vacuum and managing flow, and the impact can be just as severe as for a breastfed baby. I have seen babies who are being fed via nasogastric tube because a tongue-tie is preventing them taking milk from both breast and bottle.

In 2020 I conducted an online survey of 29 mothers who had experienced difficulties with their baby taking a bottle. Four were unable to attach to a bottle teat at all and 13 found attaching to the teat difficult. Seventeen dribbled and spilt milk while feeding, 14 struggled to manage flow and experienced gulping and choking, and 16 were troubled by wind/colic symptoms. Ten had reflux, 12 were slow to take the bottle, 13 were unable to complete full feeds due to tiring, 11 experienced slow weight gain and one baby overfed.

After division all the babies who were unable to attach to the bottle teat at all could do so, and nine of the 13 who struggled to latch could latch easily. Twelve of the 17 who dribbled milk stopped dribbling, and 11 of the 14 who gulped or choked were able to cope with the flow better. A third of the babies (five) with wind and colic improved, and half of the babies with reflux (five) showed improvement after division. Ten of the 13 who tired on the bottle were able to finish feeds and seven of the 11 with slow weight gain saw improvements in weight. For five babies the division made no difference at all. So, 82% of babies in this survey showed some improvements in feeding after tongue-tie division. It would be interesting to know what type of tongue-tie these babies had. From my own experience it is the anterior type tongue-ties that tend to cause bottle-fed babies most difficulties. Division of these in bottle-fed babies seem to result in better outcomes than division of posterior tongue-ties.

There are reports of tongue-tie impacting babies when they start on solids too. I certainly see a few babies each year who are struggling with solids. Their tongue-ties have often been previously missed because they are being bottle-fed or their mother's concerns about breastfeeding have been dismissed. The ability to lateralise the tongue seems to be crucial for babies to be able to move solid food around the mouth to aid chewing and swallowing. According to an Italian literature review by researchers at the Faculty of Dentistry, University of Cagliari (Dezio et al, 2014) a short frenulum can lead to displacement of the hyoid bone which can impact normal swallowing. They also explain how the emergence of teeth results in a shift in tongue tip position from resting between the gums to lifting higher to rest behind the upper front teeth. This shift in tongue tip position results in the cessation of tongue-thrusting seen in babies. However, a tongue-tie may prevent this change in tongue tip position and lead to a persistence of tongue-thrusting, which can be linked to babies continuing to push solids out of their mouths. However, to date, little attention has been paid to how a tongue-tie may impact solid feeding in research.

Tillie's story describes the difficulties she had with solids:

Tillie came to me at the age of six months. She was bottle-fed and had always had difficulty sustaining a seal and managing flow on the bottle. She was struggling to move food around her mouth. She had a 75% tongue-tie with no elevation and partially restricted extension and lateralisation. Her tongue looked heart shaped. After division, her mum wrote this:

'Tillie can now fully stick her tongue out, doesn't dribble or choke on her bottle and can eat solids a lot more easily. She no longer gags on the smallest amount of solids and can manage to move the food to the back of her mouth.'

The table below provides a useful summary of symptoms of tongue-tie in breast and bottle-feeding and how these relate to tongue function and first appeared in a chapter I wrote for *A Guide to Supporting Breastfeeding for the Medical Profession* (edited by Brown and Jones, 2019).

Restriction in tongue function	Symptoms
Inability to extend tongue over bottom lip	• Nipple pain and damage • Inability to latch • Difficulty latching • Difficulty sustaining the latch (baby slips down or off the breast)

Inability to lift the tongue to mid-mouth or above	• Inefficient feeding – long feeds, frequent feeds, slow weight gain, weight loss • Flow regulation issues – coughing and choking at the breast, tiring at the breast, aerophagia contributing to wind and reflux
Inability to cup the breast securely	• Difficulty sustaining the latch (baby slips down or off the breast) • Loss of suction (clicking) • Difficulty forming a seal (dribbling during feeds) • Aerophagia contributing to wind and reflux
Inability to keep the tongue in a forward position (snapback)	• Slipping off the breast • Clicking sounds during feeding
Inability to form a peristaltic wave with the tongue	• Inefficient feeding due to insufficient vacuum to transfer milk – high suck to swallow ratio, tiring, long or frequent feeds, weight issues.

Of course, these symptoms don't necessarily mean a baby has a tongue-tie. If baby has a tongue-tie, the tongue-tie may not be the only or most significant factor causing the feeding difficulties.

Nipple pain and damage – other causes

Nipple pain can be caused by multiple factors and this was found to be the case in 89% of lactation consultant consultations for nipple pain in an Australian study (Kent, 2015). By far the most common cause of nipple pain and damage is sub optimal positioning and attachment. In a study by Veronique Darmangeat which looked at 37 mothers with nipple pain, 24 of these mothers achieved comfortable feeding with adjustments to positioning and attachment. Even where a tongue-tie is contributing to a shallow, painful latch, improving positioning and attachment can help in resolving the pain and preventing further damage. Within western culture we are not brought up in environments where breastfeeding is the norm and where babies are breastfed openly and publicly, although the situation is improving with the Equality Act 2010 protecting the rights of women to breastfeed in public. Still, only 25% of UK babies are being breastfed at six months, with less than 1% still breastfeeding at one year, making UK breastfeeding rates the lowest in the world. This means new parents in the UK have very little experience or knowledge of breastfeeding, so it is a steep learning curve, with the first and most important lesson being how to position and attach the baby to the breast.

Other causes of nipple pain and damage that is difficult to heal can include infection (thrush, herpes or bacterial), vasospasm (Raynaud's Syndrome), strains in the baby's neck, jaw and cranial areas due to their position in utero (for example breech) or the birthing process, a high arched or bubble palate, flat or inverted nipples and maternal anxiety and perception of pain.

Thrush

Thrush (Candida) infection is a common infection in babies and presents as white patches in the baby's mouth, on the tongue and inside the cheeks and lips. Affected babies may also have a nappy rash which extends into the skin creases. In breastfeeding pairs, the infection can be transmitted from mother to baby or vice versa. The nipples can be red, shiny and itchy and there can sometimes be a loss of colour in the areola. However, this is not always the case and nipple pain, which often radiates deep into the breast after feeds, producing a burning or stabbing sensation, may be the only symptom.

Mothers can develop this infection secondary to antibiotic therapy, as can babies. A baby may also pick it up as they come through the birth canal if the mother is carrying the infection in her vagina. Because it is highly contagious both breasts will be affected, so nipple soreness in just one breast is not going to be due to a thrush infection. Both mum and baby need to be treated. Thrush can be difficult to differentiate from other causes of nipple pain. If the nipple looks white or is mis-shaped after feeds and mum has never had a pain-free feed, then the cause is not likely to be thrush infection. Misshaped nipples are a symptom of a shallow latch, most commonly due to sub-optimal positioning and attachment. But this nipple compression can also be the result of a tongue-tie, jaw tension or a high arched/bubble palate. Thrush can be confirmed by taking nipple and oral swabs and a nipple swab is also useful in diagnosing nipple pain caused by a bacterial infection.

Vasospasm

If a nipple looks white (blanched) after a breastfeed this is a sign of vasospasm. Vasospasm occurs when the blood supply to the nipple is compromised so the nipple turns white. Once the circulation starts to return to the nipple this can cause further colour change in the nipple. It may transition from white to purple to pink. This disturbance in circulation is accompanied by excruciating pain which radiates deep into the breast and may be described as a burning, stabbing or throbbing sensation. It is often confused with thrush infection. However, this vasospasm occurs because of Raynaud's Syndrome, a condition which affects 10% of women aged 21–50 years and is due to poor circulation in the extremities, affecting fingers, toes, and earlobes as well as nipples! It can be treated with vitamin supplements or medication.

However, vasospasm can also be secondary to a shallow

latch and compression of the nipple, so interventions to improve the latch including improving positioning and attachment and treating any tongue-tie or birth strain need to be explored before going down the medication route.

Palate shape

A palate (the roof of the mouth) which is high arched, or bubble shaped, is a common finding in babies, especially if they have a tongue-tie, as the restriction caused by the tongue-tie affects the resting posture of the tongue. When humans are relaxed and sleeping the tongue tip should elevate with the blade of the tongue contacting the roof of the mouth. This contact between the tongue and high palate helps the palate to spread. But not everyone with a high arched or bubble palate will have a tongue-tie. Genetics may be responsible in these cases. Whatever the cause, palate shape can contribute to sore nipples and difficulty sustaining the latch, which can in turn result in inefficient feeding and breast drainage. Techniques such as the exaggerated latch can be helpful in these cases. The nipple is tilted up as baby latches on so baby takes the breast tissue in high up in the mouth, filling the palate space.

A further interesting point relating to the shape of the palate and nipple pain is the fact that I often see families where babies have been diagnosed with thrush based on a white coating on the back of the tongue. This infection has been blamed for the nipple pain experienced by mum. However, the white coating on the tongue forms because the tongue does not contact the high arched palate so the dead cells on the tongue are not rubbed off and this 'rough' surface of dead cells traps milk residue. In these cases, if the tongue is wiped with a clean gauze or muslin the white coating will come off. Thrush plaques do not wipe off. This demonstrates why being supported by people skilled and knowledgeable in lactation is essential.

Flat/inverted nipples

In many cases a flat or inverted nipple will not cause issues when baby is latching and feeding at the breast. However, where babies are tongue-tied this can present a further challenge as these babies struggle to extend their tongues, form a groove and create the peristalsis (wave-like motion) to draw the nipple in to form a teat with the nipple and breast tissue. A flat or inverted nipple may not create the same stimulus for the suck reflex as a more prominent nipple does. However, even in cases where baby does not have a tongue-tie, a flat or inverted nipple which is tethered (so does not protrude when stimulated) can make latching to the breast difficult for a baby and can actually be a source of nipple pain for two reasons. First, the baby will tend to get a shallow latch as insufficient breast tissue is drawn into the mouth. Second, as the baby feeds, they will draw out the flat or inverted nipple and this stretching of the tissue can feel painful.

I remember supporting a mother several years ago who had stopped breastfeeding her first baby within the first week because her nipples were inverted. Latching and breastfeeding had been extremely painful, and her nipples had bled. When she had a second baby we agreed that she would try a nipple shield to help the baby latch more easily and to protect the nipple from trauma, as she was extremely anxious about experiencing the pain and damage she had had with her first baby. She used the shield for the first couple of weeks and in the first few days did experience some pain, but it was manageable. She then weaned her baby off the shields. Even after this relatively short period of breastfeeding the nipples had become less inverted and after six months of breastfeeding the nipples did not look inverted at all.

Flat and inverted nipples are one of the very few scenarios in which nipple shields can be helpful in establishing breastfeeding. Specific positioning and attachment techniques such as breast shaping are also helpful. This technique helps to form the breast and nipple tissue into a teat shape and makes the nipple firmer so it is easier for the baby to latch on to.

Manual stimulation prior to latching, for example rolling the nipple between your fingers, or applying suction using a breast pump or latch assist device can also be helpful. A homemade suction device can be fashioned from a 10ml syringe by cutting off the tip end and inserting the plunger in at the cut end so the smooth end will then be placed over the nipple, while the plunger is withdrawn to draw out the nipple.

Devices such as nipple formers can be worn in between or during pregnancies to help draw out a flat or inverted nipple in preparation for breastfeeding, or can also be used before feeding.

Birth interventions

Most babies I see with feeding difficulties have had a birth that has been complicated in some way. Babies born by forceps or ventouse, babies who have been breech or had another abnormal presentation, babies born by C-section, babies born with the cord around their neck and babies born after very prolonged or rapid labours are all at increased risk of feeding issues. Medication used during labour for pain relief (including epidurals) can cross the placenta and affect the baby, making them sleepy and uncoordinated with sucking in those crucial first two hours after birth. Epidurals immobilise mothers following birth, making tending to the baby and positioning them at the breast more problematic. Stitches can also make it harder for a mother to get comfortable while feeding.

A study in 2009 by Brown and Jordan (2012) which surveyed 284 mothers found that birth complications, specifically caesarean deliveries, foetal distress, failure to progress, and postpartum haemorrhage were associated with early cessation of breastfeeding for reasons of pain and difficulty. Of course where there are births involving foetal distress you are more likely to see the use of forceps and ventouse and in cases of failure to progress the artificial hormone syntocinon (or pitocin) is given to augment contractions and accelerate labour. But as Michel Odent, a French obstetrician, explains in his article on synthetic oxytocin and breastfeeding (2013), research suggests that the oxytocin receptors in the breast are desensitised by the high concentration of oxytocin given in labour and may also decrease the amount of oxytocin released by the mother during suckling. This will impair the milk ejection. Furthermore, synthetic oxytocin can also reach the baby's developing brain, and this may alter the newborn baby's feeding behaviours.

Strain and tension from birth

The pressure exerted on a baby's head by the normal contractions of labour is substantial and leads to normal head moulding (the soft bones of the skull overlap and bend) as it comes through the birth canal. When things do not go quite to plan and interventions are used, such as ventouse, forceps or caesarean section, this pressure can be prolonged or abnormally strong and lead to distortion of the bones in the skull. These babies sometimes have obvious asymmetry of the face or head. As the baby proceeds along the birth canal the head must rotate and turn and this can result in compression and strain in the neck. This abnormal head moulding and neck strain can have long-term consequences for the baby and affect their ability to latch well and feed efficiently. In these situations, referral to an osteopath, chiropractor or cranial sacral therapist can be helpful.

How birth forces can affect a baby

by Moraig Goodwin, osteopath

Entering the world is one of the most natural events in a person's life, but the actual process of childbirth is not always straightforward. As the baby descends through the birth canal she has to twist and turn to navigate a somewhat circuitous route, while at the same time being subject to the opposing forces of the mother's contractions from above and the resistance of the birth canal and cervix from below. By the time that she is born she may have experienced considerable stresses and strains in various parts of her body.

Osteopathy is a manual form of therapy which aims to remove restrictions and areas of tension in the body to allow normal movement and function to be restored. Cranial osteopathy is a very gentle form of osteopathic treatment and is particularly suitable for use on babies.

Although many of the strains and areas of tension associated with pregnancy and childbirth are thought to resolve naturally, the window of opportunity regarding establishing breastfeeding is limited. Early osteopathic intervention (whether there is a tongue-tie or not) can be an invaluable part of ensuring that a mother can make a free choice (i.e. not one dictated by considerations of pain) as to whether or not to breastfeed her baby (Hayden, 2000).

Every mother and baby's experience of childbirth is different, but there are some specific factors which can increase the chance of a baby encountering difficulties during labour:

- Positioning: *ideally a baby should be in the head-down position, facing towards the mother's back prior to the onset of labour, as this prepares her for the simplest route through the birth canal. However, if the baby's chin is not tucked in, or if she has managed to turn her head slightly* and become stuck in a bony part of the mother's pelvis, then the downward force of contractions will push her against an unyielding surface, and her spine, neck and head may absorb those forces and retain tension as a result *(Hayden, 2000, 46-8)*.

- Rapid labour: *if a baby is born very quickly, and especially if the second stage of labour (the pushing stage) is fast, then the baby is forced out, a little like the cork in a bottle of champagne! She will still have encountered the normal forces of labour but will not have had time to gently release those forces, and consequently be a little like a tightly wound spring (Hayden, 2000, 43). That tension can manifest in tightness around the jaw, neck, and shoulders (think of when you clench your jaw and hunch your shoulders when feeling stressed).*

- Slow labour: *when a baby endures contractions over a long period such as in a long labour, or where labour stops and starts, areas of tension might be more deep-rooted and therefore take longer to resolve (Hayden, 2000, 43).*

- Intervention: *when used gently, forceps and ventouse can be used to gently assist the baby in rotating as she descends through the birth canal, but often they are used at least in part to pull the baby out. The pressure required for this movement can add particular and specific strain patterns, especially around the head and neck (Hayden, 2000, 48).*

- Planned or non-emergency caesarean section: *it would be easy to think that this is the one time where these stresses should not be present, but in fact, babies have evolved to travel through the birth canal, and it is thought that the forces associated with a 'normal' birth may help to resolve any strains which were present in utero (e.g. if that baby had been in an awkward position) (Hayden, 2000, 50-1). During a planned caesarean section this does not routinely take place and so in utero strains may fail to resolve as normal.*

- Emergency caesarean section: *in this situation the baby encounters both the compressive forces of a vaginal delivery (contractions pushing from above, birth canal and cervix resisting from below) while not gaining any of the 'resolution' that it can offer (Hayden, 2000, 50-1). Also, these babies, because labour can be well established by the time that the caesarean section is decided upon, often need to be physically manhandled from deep within the mother's pelvis, and this can cause additional strain patterns to develop.*

Humans are extremely resilient, and for most babies these strain patterns and areas of tension will resolve naturally over the first few weeks of life (Hayden, 2000, 38-51). However, where they interfere with the baby's ability to breastfeed efficiently (and without pain for the mother), early osteopathic intervention can be beneficial.

Although a full-body assessment of your baby will always take place when you visit an osteopath, there are several areas which are of relevance to breastfeeding:

- *The jaw joint (known as the Temporo-Mandibular Joint or TMJ)*
- *The base of the skull*
- *The neck, upper back, and shoulders*

To establish a proper latch, the baby needs to open her mouth widely such that she can take a large portion of breast tissue (not just the mother's nipple) into her mouth (Sergueef, 2007, 277). Only when this occurs can she use her tongue to lap on the breast which stimulates the milk to flow. If the TMJ is restricted or if the associated muscles are tight, this can prove difficult. Releasing the TMJ can enable easier opening of the mouth such that the baby can establish and sustain a wide gape.

For the baby to open her mouth widely she also needs to be able to tip her head slightly backwards, thereby giving space for the jaw to open. If any of the muscles at the base of the skull are strained this movement can be difficult; releasing the tension in this area can help.

In addition, some of the muscles and nerves which are involved with tongue function are located/originate at the base of the skull (Sergueef, 2007, 275-6). Tension in this area can affect how the tongue moves. Given that tongue function is extremely important both for assisting in the draw-down of milk as well as in the transfer of milk from the front to the back of the mouth (David Elad, 2014), treatment to release tension in this area can help promote good breastfeeding technique.

Mothers often report that their baby feeds better on one side than the other. There may be a variety of reasons for this: the mother's breasts might not produce an equal supply of milk; the mother might be very one-sided and find it less comfortable to hold the baby on one side; or the baby might have a rotational or side-bending strain pattern which means that she finds it difficult to approach one breast while doing it with ease on the other. These strain patterns are often located in the neck, upper back and shoulders; releasing them can help with breastfeeding and also with helping to prevent the development of plagiocephaly (flat head syndrome), which occurs if a baby favours lying on her head in one direction (Sergueef, 2007, 95-6). Because of the proximity of the nerve centres responsible for the 'fight or flight' stress response in the upper back, osteopathic treatment of this part of the body can calm an unsettled baby, assisting with sleep patterns and thereby also helping with feeding difficulties.

Babies who have encountered trauma to the neck (for example if a tight umbilical cord is wrapped around it) can develop problems with a tiny bone in the front of the neck called the hyoid. This bone is important in tongue function owing to its muscular

45

attachments and can therefore affect tongue function adversely if affected (Sergueef, 2007, 276). Releasing the hyoid and the associated muscles can be beneficial.

Although a perfectly normal process, the forces acting upon a baby during childbirth can be considerable. While these effects mostly resolve in time, where they affect a baby's ability to breastfeed time is of the essence to ensure that the mother can make an informed and pain-free decision regarding her choice whether or not to breastfeed. Early osteopathic intervention can help to release any stresses and strains and areas of tension such that the baby can breastfeed with greater ease.

Maternal anxiety and perception of pain

In the Australian study by Kent et al (2015) 43% of women still experienced nipple pain 14 days after interventions to resolve it. We must think outside the box to understand why this might be. The focus of interventions to resolve nipple pain has tended to be on the physical causes. However, we have known for a long time that pain can be triggered or exacerbated by anxiety or depression. Indeed, when I trained as a nurse back in the late 1980s there was lots of research at the time looking at the role of anxiety in post-operative pain. The relationship between pain and anxiety and depression is complex. Chronic pain can cause depression, but pain can also be a symptom of anxiety or depression as evidenced by Means-Christensen et al (2008) in their study of primary care patients.

Many mums have depression and anxiety in the post-natal period. The NHS reports that this affects more than one in ten women. But it may go undiagnosed and undoubtedly can be a factor in chronic nipple pain. As a lactation consultant I have seen mothers who, despite our efforts to improve latch with positioning and attachment, carry out tongue-tie division and bodywork and treat nipple infections, have still not achieved pain-free feeding. As a result more of us working in infant feeding are looking at wider emotional and psychological factors and turning to other interventions to improve mental wellbeing, such as mindfulness which is something I have used in my practice with some positive results.

Anna Le Grange (Nurse, IBCLC and Mindfulness Coach) explains how relaxation techniques can be used to help with pain:

When we are in pain, our nervous system is on high alert and when we are feeling pain on a regular basis it impacts our body in many ways. We know that pain causes stress, but that stress in turn causes us to be more sensitive to pain. Thus, a negative cycle is formed. Knowing how you can break that cycle can be key to coping with ongoing pain. In an ideal world, the pain itself would be reduced, perhaps through finding a more comfortable latching position or receiving treatment from a tongue-tie practitioner or cranial osteopath. As the pain decreases you may start to feel more relaxed and less stressed. However, the memory of the pain can still be triggering in your mind before each feed. Also, many of the practical strategies can take a little time to work or get right.

Another way to interrupt the cycle is to reduce the stress. When we are stressed, we tend to tense up our body, which in turn increases the pain that we feel. By using simple relaxation techniques, we can reduce the tension in our body and calm our nervous system – our nervous system is responsible for how we feel pain and for our stress response. When we calm down our nervous system, we also slow the flow of adrenaline and cortisol which are produced from both the stress response and the pain. The good news is that it is easy to learn relaxation techniques. They are quick and simple, so perfect for when you have a new baby. Here are two simple ways that you can calm your nervous system and help your body to relax:

- *Close your eyes and put you hand on your tummy. Take 3–5 deep and slow breaths, right down into your lungs. You should feel your tummy rise on the in-breath. As you breathe out make a sigh or a whooshing sound with your breath. This is a good thing to try right before a feed.*
- *Take five minutes to listen to a short, guided relaxation. Either ask someone to be with your baby or do it when your baby is sleeping. There are lots of free apps available with short meditations. Sometimes it takes a few tries to find a voice and script that you like. You may have something from your birth preparation classes that you already like. Prioritise this every day and do it at least once. Let others who help you know how important it is to you. As time goes on you can increase the relaxation time to 10 minutes and then 15 minutes a day.*

The bonus of practising these techniques regularly is that they will also help your baby to feel more relaxed and they help the hormone oxytocin to flow, which further increases the feelings of calm relaxation and encourages your milk to flow.

Ruth Lucas et al (2018), in a randomised control trial looking at self-management of nipple pain, used cognitive behavioural exercises, deep breathing, and guided imagery. More work needs to be done on this, but what is certain is that we can modulate pain via the brain and change the experience of it. We also need to acknowledge that some people are more sensitive to pain than others and this can be influenced by genetics, as Sabu James (2013) describes in the *British Journal of Pain*. As a nurse I was taught that pain 'is whatever the patient says it is' and I believe this is where we should always start, regardless of what we see before us in terms of physical symptoms. As practitioners we have to be particularly mindful that nipple trauma and breast inflammation can have a very different appearance depending on skin colour. We won't see the redness we associate with mastitis and see on white skin if a mother has brown skin, for example. Furthermore perception of painful stimuli may be affected by sensory issues where the experience of pain will be different. In autistic parents nipple pain may be felt more acutely or not at all. Obviously both scenarios can be problematic and since pain is a warning of a problem, not feeling this sensation can lead to severe nipple trauma.

Poor weight gain – other causes

After latching difficulties and nipple pain, the other most common problem we see associated with tongue-tie is poor weight gain. A baby who is struggling to latch to the breast (or bottle) will not remove milk as effectively from the breast (or bottle) so may not receive milk in the quantities needed to grow well. However, there can be other issues affecting the transfer of milk. Palate abnormalities such as clefts can cause huge difficulties as the baby will not be able to create the necessary vacuum to draw out the milk. Babies are checked for cleft palate at their newborn and 6–8 week checks, and sometimes these abnormalities are detected on antenatal scans. However, they can be overlooked or missed, especially if the defect is subtle, so this must be kept in mind. Issues such as prematurity or low birth weight can be linked to low muscle tone, lower energy reserves and lower levels of stamina, which can lead to slower weight gain. Developmental and neurological conditions and low muscle tone can also have an impact, as well as physical abnormalities such as heart and lung conditions and laryngomalacia (floppy larynx).

Sub-optimal breastfeeding management and impact on supply

By far the most common cause of slow weight gain is sub-optimal breastfeeding management in the early days. Newborns are still often given formula top-ups to manage low blood sugars and early weight loss when mothers should be supported to express milk in these situations. Not just because the use of formula carries with it the risk of infection and can sensitise a baby to cow's milk protein, leading to allergies, but also because a lack of frequent breast stimulation and drainage in the early days is associated with longer-term impaired supply. Milk production is initially hormonally driven. High levels of the hormone progesterone in pregnancy suppress full lactation. But once the placenta comes away after birth, this progesterone level drops and triggers milk production, with milk 'coming in' at around day 3 to 4 in circumstances where mum and baby are both healthy and well, are kept together and baby has unrestricted access to the breast so feeding cues are responded to. However, birth interventions, including caesarean section, a post-partum haemorrhage, a history of hormonal disorders in the mother (such as diabetes) and separation of mother and baby may delay the onset of milk production.

Once the milk starts coming in the only thing that will establish and sustain a full supply is frequent and effective drainage of the breast, either by feeding or, if there are difficulties, by expressing (8–12 times in 24 hours). If formula is used then breastfeeding opportunities are missed, and because formula has a higher ratio of casein to whey than breastmilk, it will fill a baby up for longer so they will ask to be fed less frequently. So, even if they are put to the breast at every feed and then topped up with formula, feeding frequency will be reduced, to the detriment of supply. So it is far better to express after offering the breast and top-up with expressed breastmilk.

Because we have a bottle-feeding culture, I find many parents are surprised by the number of times a baby needs to feed. Babies have small stomachs and big growth needs so they need to feed little and often. Babies fed formula not only feed less often, but the use of a bottle also often leads to overfeeding as the flow is faster than at the breast and parents often feel pressured to ensure babies take set amounts and finish feeds, even if the baby is showing signs of being satisfied. This further reduces feeding frequency. It is not unusual for me to see parents with babies of just 3–5 days old who have been told to give 50–60ml top-ups, which is more than a breastfed baby would take at a full feed. Inevitably many of these babies are sick after feeds, adding to anxieties about whether they are getting enough.

When babies are struggling to get what they need directly from the breast, regularly expressing at least 8 to 10 times per day, starting as soon as possible and within the first six hours after birth is imperative, but is often overlooked. If a mum can establish and maintain a full milk supply it buys us time to sort out the latching issues, divide any tongue-tie and so on. There is nothing more disheartening for me and more heart-breaking for parents than when I see a baby who is six weeks old and mum has been expressing 2–3 times a day and is getting around 100ml of expressed milk in 24 hours. That is a very tough situation to rescue. While supply can still be increased at this stage, it is a slow process involving high levels of commitment and it is less likely a mum will get to a full supply if she never established one in the first place. When feeding is going well mothers will produce around 500ml in 24 hours by the end of the first week after birth, and by day 14 this will be up to around 750ml. Milk supply is established within the first 3–6 weeks. The older the baby gets, the harder it is to increase supply. Those early days are crucial. Feeding and/or expressing 8–12 times in 24 hours is hard work, but it is an investment in the long term and makes for a much easier breastfeeding journey.

Hormonal disorders and breast surgery
Hormonal disorders such as diabetes, thyroid issues and

polycystic ovary syndrome (PCOS) can impact on milk supply, particularly if they are not well controlled in the case of diabetes and hypothyroidism. But another factor that is often overlooked in cases of slow weight gain or weight loss in relation to low milk supply is a history of breast surgery. Breast reduction surgery can involve the removal of some of the glandular tissue (the milk factory), damage to milk ducts and nerve severing (particularly if the nipples have been removed and re-sited). This can have a negative impact on production and the ability to breastfeed, but in these cases I would always advise seeking help from an IBCLC in pregnancy and having a plan in place to optimise milk production afterwards, as many mothers who have had reduction surgery can and do go on to breastfeed with the right help and support. Breast implants are generally less problematic if the nerves to the nipples have not been damaged and it is better if the implant has been placed beneath the muscle, as is common practice. However, this depends on the reason for the implants. Breast enhancement simply to increase a cup size is not likely to be a significant issue. But if you never developed breasts at puberty and had implants for that reason you may not produce more than a few drops of milk. Nature has played a cruel trick and not provided you with the glandular tissue needed.

Insufficient glandular tissue

The lack of breast development in puberty can come in varying degrees and the markers for a condition called insufficient glandular tissue (IGT), also known as mammary hypoplasia, can include very small, flat breasts, tubular shaped breasts, significant breast asymmetry with one breast being much larger than the other, a large gap between the breasts and a lack of breast changes during puberty and pregnancy. My own view on this is that breasts should be checked in pregnancy so any problems such as this can be identified, and a plan put in place to optimise milk production. Most mothers in this situation will be able to breastfeed, but milk production may be compromised and their babies need close monitoring to ensure they are getting enough. Unfortunately, all too often this is a problem that is picked up only after several weeks of concerns about weight gain and milk supply and only then if the mother sees a knowledgeable IBCLC.

Reflux and colic – other causes

Reflux and colic issues are most certainly associated with tongue-tie. A study by American Oral Surgeon Scott Siegel (2016) found that symptoms resolved in half of the 1,000 babies he treated for tongue-tie. A further study (Slagter et al, 2020) also concluded that tongue-tie division can resolve reflux problems. Tongue-tie may contribute to reflux symptoms due to the intake of air because of a poor seal on the breast or bottle, and difficulties regulating flow. But there may be other causes of reflux which can coexist alongside a tongue-tie or occur in babies without a tongue-tie. These include a weak lower oesophageal sphincter (stomach valve) which allows milk to be regurgitated back up from the stomach, cow's milk protein allergy, overfeeding in bottle-fed babies and over-supply in breastfed babies. In babies with a weak lower oesophageal sphincter, symptoms will usually resolve within the first year of life as tone in the sphincter improves. This is probably the most common cause of spit up in babies and these babies are often termed 'happy spitters', as in many cases it doesn't cause them any discomfort or affect weight gain. In the case of cow's milk protein allergy there are usually other symptoms such as skin rashes, nasal congestion and mucous and/or blood in the stools, which may also be green, and these babies are often in discomfort. Overfeeding in bottle-fed babies can be resolved simply by reducing feed volumes so babies feed little and often, and using paced bottle-feeding techniques. Oversupply is more commonly seen in mothers who have previously breastfed and sometimes in mothers who have had a premature or sick baby and have done a lot of expressing in the early days. The force of the milk ejection reflex ('let down') can be overwhelming in this situation and these babies can come off the breast coughing and choking at the start of feeds. They will sometimes attempt to slow the flow by breaking the seal and you can hear a clicking sound when they do this. The intake of air, alongside difficulty managing the forceful milk flow, can trigger regurgitation/ reflux and tummy discomfort. Strategies such as expressing off the initial let down (around 30ml) before offering the breast, more upright or laid-back feeding positions to slow the flow and block feeding can be used to manage oversupply and an easy way to reduce reflux is to keep baby upright for 20–30 minutes after feeds.

All of these factors mean that we should never assume that impairment in tongue function, difficulty latching, and inefficient feeding is simply due to a restricted lingual frenulum, as that can lead to over treatment with poor outcomes. It is important to consider the whole picture, as even in the presence of a tongue-tie there may be other issues affecting feeding that need addressing. For these reasons, a robust feeding assessment carried out by healthcare professionals with advanced feeding knowledge and skills is especially important. A multidisciplinary approach involving an IBCLC, a medic (paediatrician and/or ENT surgeon), a speech and language therapist and a body worker (perhaps a physio or occupational therapist, or an osteopath) would be a gold standard for the tackling more complex difficulties. Sadly, our current systems mean that this sort of collaboration rarely occurs.

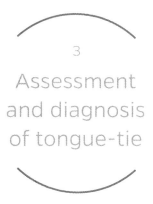

3

Assessment and diagnosis of tongue-tie

Difficulties in identifying a tongue-tie

In the first chapter I discussed why the issue of tongue-tie and its impact on infant feeding is overlooked and why it can be so challenging to get it recognised. In the second chapter we explored some of the difficulties we have in defining what a tongue-tie is and how thinking has changed on this, especially in terms of the anatomy. In this context it is not surprising that parents can find themselves caught up in confusing information and terminology, and conflicting opinions.

So how do practitioners who divide tongue-ties go about deciding if a baby has a tongue-tie which is impacting on feeding and if that baby is likely to benefit from having a division? I would firstly say, without any apology, that I firmly believe that babies should not be undergoing division for feeding issues unless they have been reviewed by an IBCLC or someone with equivalent knowledge, training, experience and skills. How you ascertain that somebody has this knowledge, training, experience, and skills if they have not gone through the accreditation process set by the International Board of Lactation Consultant Examiners, I am not sure. It is extremely disappointing that the UK UNICEF Baby Friendly Initiative and the NHS continue to fail to recognise the role and value of the IBCLC. Fortunately, parents are becoming more aware of their value, which can only be a good thing.

My reason for insisting on input from an IBCLC is because, as discussed in the last chapter, breastfeeding difficulties arise for a multitude of reasons and other challenges often exist alongside a tongue-tie or are overlooked because of concerns about a tongue-tie. When this happens, we are in danger of over-diagnosing, over-treating and failing to provide the right support to help parents successfully feed their babies. It concerns me greatly when I see referral pathways for division which involve referrals being made by healthcare professionals (be they midwives, health visitors or GPs) with minimal or no specific training in infant feeding and tongue-tie assessment. These babies are then seen for 20 minutes in a hospital outpatient department by a surgeon, again with no specific training in infant feeding or tongue-tie assessment, and a decision is then made on whether to divide or not. Sometimes the right decision is made. But I see many babies who have been declined a division who desperately needed one. These decisions often focus on the baby's weight gain with feeding being deemed satisfactory purely because the baby is gaining weight. However, no account is taken of the quality of the feeding experience. A baby may be struggling to sustain the latch at the breast, be suffering with excessive wind or reflux, and be working excessively hard just to get enough milk to sustain himself. The mother may have nipple pain and damage and be in agony every time baby feeds. Or she may be having to pump several times per day to top her baby up to sustain adequate weight gain. Breastfeeding must work for both mother and baby. It should not be an endurance test.

Just as worryingly, I am seeing increasing numbers of babies who have been referred by midwives and infant feeding leads for division of a 'very posterior tongue-tie'. Other factors which are impacting the tongue function and feeding have been completely overlooked and there is not a frenulum that needs dividing. This issue has increased with growing awareness among healthcare professionals. When study days on just the basics are offered to midwives and health visitors, staff may go away thinking they have the necessary skills to diagnose a tongue-tie and present themselves as 'specialists' to parents.

I have been fortunate to be involved in training health visitors in Kent in identifying potential tongue-ties. But they are clear that their role is to identify potential signs and symptoms. They then refer to a specialist clinic where the mother and baby have a much more thorough assessment with an IBCLC before any decision about a referral for division is made. This to me seems like a very sensible and safe approach.

Learning to assess tongue function and diagnose tongue-tie takes many days of training and many months of experience. I have done hundreds of hours of training and I train others. I have assessed in the region of 10,000 babies and performed divisions in over 4,000 babies over an 11-year period. Still I question my decisions, have doubts, and seek advice from colleagues about some of the more complex feeding situations I see.

So how are tongue-ties assessed?

The place to start with assessment of tongue-tie is to look at feeding. For breastfeeding to work the single most important issue is the latch. Most breastfeeding difficulties will stem from a sub-optimal latch. In the early 1990s a tool was developed by Deborah Jenson and colleagues based on the acronym LATCH which looked at how well a baby latches, how much audible swallowing is evident, nipple type, mother's comfort level and how much help the mother needs with holding the baby.

This tool is still used today in practice and in research and highlights the key areas of interest when observing breastfeeding. In addition, when assessing latch we need to look at the 'suck to swallow ratio', as this tells us a lot about the efficiency of the baby at the breast. A ratio of 1–3 sucks per swallow is considered normal. But I see babies who may be taking anything from 4–30 sucks per swallow! A baby taking so many sucks in order to remove a mouthful of milk to swallow is working very hard, will tire quickly and will end up feeding constantly or frequently, usually with very short bursts of sucking and swallowing and lots of pauses. These are the babies that never appear settled and satisfied and need constant stimulation to keep them feeding. They spend many hours on the breast, but this is not reflected in their weight gain. A baby spending many hours at the breast should be gaining above expectations. These babies often struggle to gain enough weight.

So the feeding pattern also needs to be assessed. This is controversial and has the power to polarise breastfeeding counsellors, lactation consultants and healthcare professionals. Nils J. Bergman (2013), a Swedish public health physician specialising in perinatal neuroscience, writes:

> There is insufficient evidence on optimal neonatal feeding intervals, with a wide range of practices. The stomach capacity could determine feeding frequency. A literature search was conducted for studies reporting volumes or dimensions of stomach capacity before or after birth. Six articles were found, suggesting a stomach capacity of 20ml at birth. A stomach capacity of 20ml translates to a

feeding interval of approximately 1h for a term neonate. This corresponds to the gastric emptying time for human milk, as well as the normal neonatal sleep cycle.

Sleep cycles in newborns are around 45 minutes in length. So, what we find in babies in the early weeks of life is that they can be very frequent feeders.

The UNICEF Breastfeeding Assessment Tools talk about babies in the early weeks needing a minimum of 8–12 breastfeeds in 24 hours with feeding durations of 5–40 minutes regarded as normal. However, this is often seen by parents, and indeed some healthcare professionals, as 'excessive'. This is because in the UK and most of the western world formula feeding is still the cultural norm. But the feeding pattern we see in a formula fed baby is not going to reflect the biological norm, which is the breastfed baby, for several reasons.

Firstly, formula milk has a much longer gastric emptying time. In a study from 1981 (Cavell, 1981) which looked at 17 healthy babies aged four weeks to six months they found that the average gastric half-emptying time for meals of human breast milk was 48 minutes, compared to 78 minutes for infant formula. The higher casein to whey ratio in formula milk contributes to the longer gastric emptying time. Secondly, we know that bottle-feeding tends to lead to bigger volumes being taken at each feed (Hester et al, 2012), with studies demonstrating that formula-fed babies take in significantly greater amounts of energy and protein (66–70% more protein in a study by Heisnig et al, 1993).

There is little information provided to parents on appropriate milk volumes, and the amount a baby needs does increase in the first month of life. Formula packaging tends to encourage parents to give larger volumes to reduce the number of feeds and add to the 'convenience' of formula feeding. Let's face it, if you are going to have to wash and sterilise bottles, and boil a kettle to make up formula safely (as per NHS guidelines) 12 times per day, breastfeeding, with safe fresh milk at the right temperature on tap, is the much easier option.

Another factor that can influence the frequency of feeding in a breastfed baby is breast storage capacity (Mohrbacher, 2011). This is the amount of storage space available for milk within the glandular (milk-producing) tissue of the breast. It is unrelated to breast size. But a mother with a larger milk storage capacity will find her baby can go longer between feeds than a mother with a smaller storage capacity. As a breast becomes full milk production slows down and milk then needs to be promptly removed to maintain adequate milk production. With a larger storage capacity, it takes longer for the breast to fill and for a reduction in production to be triggered so feeding intervals can be longer without impacting on supply. However, as storage capacity is unrelated to breast size there is no way of predicting how much storage capacity a mother has. So, feeding in every situation needs to be baby-led. However, if you find that your baby is feeding less or more often than your friends' baby, but both babies are thriving, this may be an explanation.

Despite the fact we have an obesity problem in the developed world, with 2.4% of children aged 4–5 in the UK being severely obese in 2017–2018, one of the biggest concerns parents have is whether their babies are 'getting enough'. This leads to unfounded concerns about milk supply, weight gain and feeding patterns and unnecessary topping up and over-feeding. Both parents and the professionals supporting them need an understanding of what is normal in terms of feeding pattern, what can influence this and when there is need for concern.

I have colleagues in the world of lactation, be they IBCLCs, breastfeeding counsellors or peer supporters, who are what

I term the 'tongue-tie doubters'. They do not accept that tongue-ties are ever an issue. Many promote the idea that all breastfeeding issues can be 'fixed' with positioning and attachment techniques, practice, and perseverance on the part of the mother.

Breastfeeding is certainly a learned skill. This learning is not made any easier for many of us because we simply have not been brought up around breastfeeding mothers and babies. Before learning to drive a car or ride a bike most of us have already seen others do it. We already know where the accelerator pedal is on the car and that pressing it makes the car go faster. We know that we need to hold the handlebars on a bike to steer. How many new parents have held a baby before they hold their own, or feel confident handling a baby? How many know how to hold a baby at the breast?

Invariably, when I ask parents in antenatal sessions to show me how they will hold the baby at the breast, they place the doll with its head in the crook of their arm, flat on its back looking up towards the ceiling. This is a bottle-feeding position, and it is our 'go to' reference for feeding a baby because it is what we are familiar with. Learning how to hold and position baby at the breast and attach them to the breast effectively will take a bit of time and we will not always get it right. However, with practice and help it should start to become easier within days and be second nature within weeks.

Using nipple soreness and damage as an example, as this is the most common difficulty associated with tongue-tie, some nipple soreness in the early days may be part of the learning process. But we should not be seeing mothers with severe nipple pain and damage in the early days or with nipple pain and damage that persists for weeks or months. For mothers and babies with persistent breastfeeding issues we must look beyond positioning and attachment and stop telling them to 'power through'. Breastfeeding should not be so hard! It is a normal activity for mammals and one upon which the survival of the species depends.

Vicky Barbour Andrews, who runs 'The Baby Experts' directory in Suffolk, wrote this in a blog published on her website www.thebabyexpertsuffolk.co.uk:

As my baby was crying, I noticed the good old tell-tale sign of tongue-tie as the tip of her tongue was heart-shaped. My thoughts of tongue-tie were dismissed and I continued to attempt to breastfeed. Eventually the midwives left, and we were left to fend for ourselves with the promise that the breastfeeding lady would swing by the following day on her way into work.

That night quite simply was hell, Hattie screamed all night and would latch and unlatch constantly.

The breastfeeding lady arrived as promised the following morning and tried to get Hattie to latch on, she would for a while but as had been the story all night would unlatch without managing a full feed and she was getting increasingly fraught.

I mentioned to the breastfeeding lady that my nipple looked like a lipstick after Hattie had fed and that this was a sign of tongue tie but again that notion was dismissed.

I persevered, constantly doubting myself. Surely the midwives and the breastfeeding lady must know what to look for.

At Hattie's 3-day checks she had lost 7.9% of her birth weight and my nipples resembled something out of a horror movie. We were told to go and see a midwife again a few days later to check on her weight loss but when we did the midwife we saw dismissed everything and said we were just off the guideline loss of 8% so not to worry about it.

By this point I was in so much pain every time I attempted to breastfeed that I was beginning to dread attempting to feed Hattie. Every time she latched on I had to count loudly up to 10 to try and distract myself from the pain.

Unfortunately this started to affect my mental health. I was beating myself up about how me as a new mum would not want to feed her beautiful baby, how I was filled with dread every time Hattie started fussing for a feed, how could I not be filled with joy at that beautiful thing that breastfeeding is.

I have suffered from depression historically and I work extremely hard to stay on top of my mental health, I know that once I hit a certain point there's no stopping it and it takes over.

At this point I felt there was no option but to stop breastfeeding and to move to bottle-feeding. Bottle feeding was no easier for Hattie and she still suffered with everything a tongue-tie baby does so I booked an appointment to see a private tongue-tie practitioner who confirmed Hattie had a tongue-tie and separated it for us.

Any feeding assessment needs to consider what compensations a mother is having to use to manage any nipple pain or damage and to ensure her baby is 'getting enough' to grow and develop. I see mothers who tell me that feeding is only tolerable if they feed in one position. Often that position involves contortions for both mum and baby: the use of pillows, the need to constantly hold the breast in the baby's mouth to stop them slipping, the use of nipple shields and sometimes regular analgesia. We must ask ourselves whether the help we have provided has worked. If it has not, it is not good enough to tell mothers to 'put up with it' and 'power through'. We need to do more, and for parents this may mean finding alternative means of support.

Amy Linthicum-Watson shares her experience of a missed tongue-tie on her blog: www.minbodymamatulsa.com.

Nursing was awkward, and I kept forgetting to keep her tummy to tummy. Positions did not feel organic. Kaylen didn't have much quiet, alert time. She was either sleeping or crying to nurse or at the breast. I had the hospital lactation consultant come to my room several times to make sure I had it down before going home but despite my best efforts by the second day my nipples were bleeding. I was given lanolin and a nipple shield and sent on my way. At our first paediatrician appointment, Kaylen had lost 13% of her birth weight. I was devastated. She nursed all the time! I was in terrible pain and barely sleeping. The on-staff LC came in and gave me the first of many talks about supplementing with formula. I began sobbing uncontrollably.

Having assessed feeding the next step is to assess tongue function to see if this is impaired and then to establish if this is due to a restricted lingual frenulum (tongue-tie).

During a feeding assessment a feed will usually be observed and this forms part of the assessment of tongue function. When watching a baby latch to the breast we expect to see the tongue coming down and forward and forming a groove as baby latches. We expect the baby to stay securely latched at the breast. Any slipping, or loss of seal and suction characterised by clicking sounds tells us there may be an issue with tongue function. Lots of short sucking bursts, frequent pausing, infrequent swallowing and falling asleep tells us baby is working hard to create the vacuum to draw the milk. Gulping and choking tells us there is an issue with managing the flow.

All these observations give us clues about tongue function.

When looking at tongue function we have a choice of tools to use. The most well-known, oldest, and most widely used is the Hazelbaker Assessment Tool for Lingual Frenulum Function (HATLFF). This was developed by American IBCLC Dr Alison Hazelbaker in 1992. Crucially it looks at function as well as appearance. The assessment is scored on seven functions: elevation, extension, lateralisation, cupping, peristalsis, snap back and spread of the front part of the tongue; and five appearance items: appearance of the tongue tip when lifted, elasticity of the frenulum, length of the frenulum and where the frenulum attached to the tongue and where it attaches to the lower gum. Each item is scored, and these scores determine whether the tongue function and frenulum are normal or whether division is indicated. Babies with borderline scores may respond well to conservative approaches and will not all need division. The tool was found to have high reliability in a study by Amir et al (2006). The researchers also noted that function could be more simply assessed using just the three functions of lateralisation, extension and elevation. This information has been utilised in the development of other assessment tools since.

One of the criticisms of the Hazelbaker Tool is that it is difficult to use. It does require training, and as a trademarked tool the training must be provided by Alison Hazelbaker herself or someone authorised by her. So other tools have been developed. These include the Bristol Tongue Assessment Tool (Ingram et al, 2016) and its pictorial version, The Tongue-tie and Breastfed Babies Assessment Tool (Ingram et al, 2019), the Neonatal Tongue Screening Test (Lopez de Castro Martinelli, 2016) and the Frenotomy Decision Tool for Breastfeeding Dyads (Srinivasan, Dobrich et al, 2006).

The Bristol Tongue Assessment Tool (BTAT) and The

Tongue-tie and Breastfed Babies Assessment Tool (TABBY) are basically much shorter versions of the HATLFF. They consist of just four items: tongue extension, tongue elevation, tongue tip appearance and attachment of the frenulum to the gum. Scores are out of eight, with scores of 6–7 being borderline and scores of five or under indicating a restriction which may be affecting feeding. The team that developed these tools reports a strong and significant correlation with the HATLFF (Ingram et al, 2016). However, a study comparing the BTAT with the Neonatal Tongue Screening Test (which looks at lip posture, elevation of tongue during crying, tongue shape when lifted, frenulum thickness and visibility, and frenulum attachment to the tongue and the floor of the mouth) found that the Neonatal Tongue Screening Test (NTST) was more effective in determining breastfeeding difficulties. A prevalence of tongue-tie of 2.6% was picked up by the Bristol Tool compared to 11.7% with the NTST. However, both tools have undergone validation studies and are regarded as reliable. I would suggest that the discrepancies arise from the fact that the Bristol Tool only consists of four items, whereas the NTST and HATLFF encompass a broader range of appearance and functional indicators of tongue-tie so could be expected to be more sensitive.

I have not been able to identify any validation studies relating to the Frenotomy Decision Tool by Carole Dobrich. This tool is in three sections. The first relates to breastfeeding and includes items on nipple pain, latch, efficiency, and weight gain. The second section looks at tongue function (extension, lateralisation, elevation, and cupping) and oral anatomy (the presence of a white-coated tongue, which can be associated with tongue-tie), with the third section looking at lip tie. I like the fact that this tool incorporates feeding issues. However, including a section which evaluates lip tie is problematic given the lack of evidence that lip ties have an impact on infant feeding. This is something that is discussed further in Chapter 6.

While the tools developed in Bristol (BTAT and TABBY) are easy to teach and learn and are helpful in identifying potential tongue-ties, my own preference is to use the HATLFF. This is because this tool incorporates items which assess sucking. This can be extremely useful information to have in terms of explaining how the tongue is impacting feeding and in identifying other factors which may potentially be contributing, such as poor muscle tone, coordination issues and jaw tension. This information is also extremely helpful in anticipating and supporting any difficulties which may arise or continue after division.

Some practitioners choose not to use a tool, with some just assessing lateralisation, elevation and extension and the appearance of the frenulum. However, the use of a tool seems to me to be good practice as it can provide a quantifiable measure of tongue function and helps in documenting the appearance of the tongue and frenulum. Using a tool is helpful when discussing the decision to divide with parents as the scores provide an objective way of evaluating any impact the lingual frenulum is having. Parents are not just being given the practitioner's opinion.

A video of an assessment of tongue function can be found on my website sarahoakleylactation.co.uk/tongue-tie-assessment-and-division-services as well as the assessment tools mentioned here.

The difference between and anterior and posterior tongue-tie

Parents often get confused by the way practitioners describe their baby's tongue-tie. Some parents are told their baby has a 'posterior' tongue-tie, some are told it is 'anterior', and some are told it is both. These terms describe the appearance of the lingual frenulum. They do not tell us anything about function, which is what treatment decisions need to be based on. An anterior tongue-tie is where the frenulum is attached close to the tip of the tongue. A posterior tongue-tie is where the frenulum is attached further back along the under-surface of the tongue.

But how far back? This is a subject of controversy. Many argue that a true posterior tongue-tie would be the sub-mucosal type tongue-tie which was first defined in 2004 by Catherine Watson Genna as a thick band of tissue under the mucosa (lining of the mouth). However, the new research on anatomy (Mills et al, 2019) has demonstrated that tongue-ties are not a band of tissue, and there is no band of tissue at the base of the tongue under the mucosa. So this concept is now being rejected in favour of the idea that the tension which can be felt at the base of the tongue, in some babies who show restriction in tongue function, is in fact due to muscular tension. This may be triggered by the baby's position in the womb or trauma and strain from the process of birth.

There is also evidence that the tension felt at the base of the tongue may be due to a shortening of the genioglossus muscle (situated at the base of the tongue) and this shortening may occur alongside a tongue-tie or on its own (Ferres-Amat E et al, 2016). As someone who divides tongue-ties this makes sense to me as sometimes, after releasing a tongue-tie, the base of the tongue still feels tense, but there is no further frenulum to divide. I would speculate that the lack of mobility of the tongue in utero, caused by a tight frenulum, may contribute to the shortening of the genioglossus muscle. Tongue function may improve in these situations. But some restriction may still be evident. Ferres-Amat E et al (2016) describe using the more radical division method of Z-plasty (described in Chapter 5) combined with myotomy (release of the genioglossus muscle) in children aged 4–14 with impaired speech and dental issues.

Other surgeons, such as Dr Soroush Zaghi, a US ENT and sleep surgeon, uses a similar approach when dividing tongue-ties in older children and adults.

In the literature any tongue-tie where the frenulum is attached halfway or further back along the under-surface of the tongue is referred to as 'posterior'. Catherine Watson Genna and others refer to 'types' of tongue ties. These equate to a classification system developed by Mervyn Griffiths (2004) which uses percentages to describe the appearance of a tongue-tie. So, a tongue-tie referred to as 'type one' would be a '100%' tongue tie (attached to the tongue tip and therefore anterior). A 'type 2' would be 75% (attached a quarter of the way back from the tongue tip and still anterior). A 'type 3' would be 50% or less (attached halfway back or more from the tongue tip and generally defined as posterior).

The most important thing to remember is that is does not matter what type of tongue-tie your baby has. It is how the tongue-tie affects the function of the tongue and thus feeding which is important.

Ask the healthcare professional who is seeing your baby for tongue-tie division how they are assessing your baby. What are they looking at in terms of function of the tongue? How does the function relate to the feeding problems you are experiencing? Which assessment tool are they using and what are the scores? What do those scores indicate? How have they reached their opinion on whether your baby needs a division? What outcome do they hope to achieve from division? If they do not believe your feeding issues are due to a tongue-tie, can they explain why you are struggling, how to resolve the problems and direct you to further help and support? Don't be embarrassed to ask these questions because you, your baby and your feeding journey matter. It matters that you are comfortable with the information you are being given.

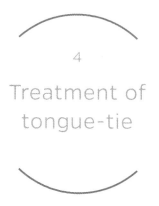

4

Treatment of tongue-tie

There are three procedures that can be used for dividing tongue-ties:

- *Frenulotomy* (referred to as frenotomy in the USA) is the simplest. It involves making a simple incision in the frenulum to 'divide' it, releasing the tension the frenulum is creating to free up tongue movement. Scissors are most often used, but a scalpel can be used too. This procedure is minimally invasive, quick and can be done without the use of local or general anaesthetics.
- *Frenectomy* is a procedure which involves the removal of the frenulum. This can be done using a blade or scissors to completely excise the frenulum and sutures are placed. This procedure usually requires a general anaesthetic in babies and young children but can be done under local anaesthetic in older children and adults. Laser and electro cautery can also be

used to perform frenectomy. These methods remove the frenulum by vapourising the frenula tissue and suturing is not needed. Both can be done without the need for general anaesthetic, although local anaesthetic is usually used.

- *Z-plasty* involves the surgical removal of the frenulum and the creation of opposing triangular flaps which are sutured to allow free movement of the tongue. This is quite an involved procedure and, like frenectomy, is usually done under a general anaesthetic in young children.

Frenulotomy with scissors is the most commonly used procedure for division of tongue-tie in babies under one. It is simple to teach and learn, involves minimal equipment and no drugs. It can be done in community settings by a single practitioner and is therefore cheap to provide. Baby is wrapped in a blanket and the parent or other helper holds baby's head still. The tongue is lifted up with the practitioner's index finger (sometimes an index and middle finger may be used, or a Brodie director which is a grooved spade-shaped instrument) and the frenulum is divided with the scissors. I use curved, blunt-tipped strabismus scissors, but some of my colleagues use other types of scissors according to their own preferences. I prefer blunt tips as this helps me to judge how far back to divide and I do not have to be concerned about catching other surrounding structures, which may be a risk with pointed-tip scissors.

The procedure takes just seconds and the baby is fed immediately afterwards. Babies tolerate it well as it is an extremely quick procedure and because sutures are not used there is less discomfort afterwards, so babies are less likely to struggle with feeding or develop oral aversion, and there is a lower risk of infection. The main issues with frenulotomy are recurrence and bleeding.

Recurrence

Our understanding of why tongue-ties recur is still developing. Recurrences do happen, even after the more radical procedures of frenectomy and Z-plasty. In some cases, it is likely that the wound edges simply adhere back together again. Most of us who divide have occasionally seen babies where within a few days the tongue-tie has recurred and looks almost as if it were never divided in the first place, even when we know full division took place. Scarring certainly seems to be an issue. My own thoughts on this are that as the wound heals and forms a scar there are cases where this scar tissue becomes excessively thick and/or tight. This then causes a restriction in the way the tongue can move and essentially forms what looks like and behaves like another 'tongue-tie'. This explains why parents talk about the 'tongue-tie growing back'.

Until the first study on frenula anatomy was published in 2014 it was thought that the lingual frenulum was composed of mucous membrane (mucosa). Alison Hazelbaker wrote in 2010 in her book *Tongue-tie: Morphogenesis, Impact, Assessment and Treatment,* 'Scar tissue formation that further impairs tongue function seems to be unsupported in the literature and appears to be an unreasonable concern… the tissue of the mouth rarely even forms scar tissue… Mucosa is flexible enough to withstand traction, so scar tissue has much less opportunity to form. A scar would form only if the tissue remained relatively immobile'. However, we now know that the frenulum can be composed of three layers (mucosa, fascia, and muscle). Those of us who divide have always observed that the thicker frenula seem to be the ones that are most likely to require re-division. These thicker frenula were found, in the Brazilian study of 2014, to contain collagen fibres, which predispose to scarring. The more recent New Zealand studies (Mills et al, 2019) have confirmed the involvement of fascia and muscle and fascia is primarily composed of collagen so can be expected to scar as it heals.

So, does this mean that any tongue-tie which is thicker and involves the fascial layer will inevitably require re-division and may not have a successful outcome? The answer to that is most definitely 'no'. While we do not have any specific studies on the causes of recurrence of tongue-tie, we know that the appearance of the frenulum only tells us a small part of the story. A further study by the Mills team (Mills et al, 2020) on the histology of the lingual frenulum reports that there is significant individual variability in the proportions and distribution of collagen and elastin fibres which will influence the properties of the fascia and potentially have an impact on the range of tongue function. This variability does not seem to relate to age. Obviously, the composition and flexibility of the fascia, which after all extends across the whole floor of the mouth, may influence the degree of mobility achieved post-division, as well as any scarring.

When dividing tongue-ties I certainly find some are more 'fibrous' in texture than others and these are not always the thicker looking tongue-ties. Some of the thicker ones are very soft in texture. My assumption is that the more fibrous the frenulum feels, the more likely it is that we will have an issue with recurrence. But babies with 'soft' ones do sometimes come back with ongoing feeding issues and have recurrence, and the more fibrous ones don't always.

Is there anything we can do about this issue of recurrence? From my own experience I have found that babies who breastfeed frequently after division tend to do better. But this could be for a number of reasons. It could be that the regular movement of the tongue helps to reduce contracture of the wound, which is a normal part of wound healing, and perhaps this helps with reducing the risk of tight scarring. It could also be that babies who feed frequently post-division are developing the tongue muscle, and this leads to better feeding outcomes. Certainly, those babies who can feed frequently will be getting lots of practice and stimulating milk supply and both things will help achieve better feeding outcomes, whatever the breastfeeding challenge. Tightness in the fascia, muscles and other soft tissues throughout the head and neck area may also be released to a degree by this frequent feeding.

In addition to keeping the tongue mobile through frequent feeding, myself and many of my colleagues recommend simple exercises such as finger-sucking, tongue-poking games and eliciting lateral movement by running the tip of an index finger along baby's lower gum and back again so the tongue tip follows. These exercises are included in the After-Care Advice Sheet produced by the UK-based Association of Tongue-tie Practitioners.

If you do your own research via the internet on tongue-tie it is likely you will quickly find information and discussions on recurrence and its prevention. It is an emotive topic as no parent or practitioner wants to see babies going through multiple procedures and no one wants to see parents and babies continuing to struggle with feeding issues.

Disruptive wound massage

Disruptive wound massage (DWM) and wound stretches are interventions which have been advocated now for several years. However, it is important to understand that there is no evidence base to demonstrate that this approach is safe and effective and there have been lots of concerns about the associated risks. These approaches have been most popular among US and Australian-based practitioners, with only a handful in the UK recommending them.

The theory behind these approaches derives from what we know about how wounds heal. As a wound heals, the edges, which are in close apposition, knit together. I am using the word 'knit' because it captures the complex nature of wound healing which involves three stages: inflammation, proliferation, and maturation. The inflammatory phase is the initial phase involving bleeding, clotting and the delivery of nutrients and oxygen to begin tissue repair and white cells and antibodies to prevent infection. The proliferation phase is where damaged cells form fibroblasts which serve as bridges allowing cells to migrate round the wound and secrete collagen which will form into fibres across the wound and create new tissue known as granulation tissue (the knitting bit). The wound will then contract and get slowly smaller as the skin layer, or in the case of tongue-tie the mucosa, forms. In the maturation phase the wound is closed and goes through a process of remodelling during which time any scarring will regress. The remodelling stage can take up to two years and the wound area will remain weaker than it was pre-surgery or injury.

DWM and stretches aim to impact healing at the proliferation stage by slowing down the process of wound contraction and closure. They are often compared to the established practice of healing by secondary intention. 'Healing by secondary intention' is the term applied when you have a deep wound that is forming a cavity or sinus. We do not want this type of wound to heal over with new skin too quickly, as this can leave a cavity underneath which can be a site for infection and lead to further wound breakdown. Packs may be inserted into these wounds to stop the edges coming together too quickly before formation of granulation tissue, to fill the space from the bottom up, has taken place. However, a tongue-tie division wound should not be leaving a deep cavity to be filled and at some point the wound edges will have to come together. There will be wound contracture and a scar will form. Delaying this process by reopening the wound with massage or stretches may increase the risk of scarring, and therefore recurrence, because it can prolong the inflammatory phase of healing. Papathanasiou et al 2017 write that 'many studies support the contribution of dysregulated, exaggerated inflammation in scar formation'.

This is one mother's experience of disruptive wound massage:

Following a second division after the first division was unsuccessful and the tongue-tie recurred I was willing to try anything the second time round. I appreciated that there was no evidence wound management provided a better outcome, but equally there is no evidence to suggest that it has an adverse effect so I thought I had nothing to lose by doing it. It was done on the advice of the practitioner who divided the tongue-tie. For the first week, every morning and evening we undertook firm massage of the wound by applying pressure with our index finger and slowly moving it round in a small circle (within the diamond) for six seconds. The aim was to move the four edges of the diamond apart. For the next five weeks, we massaged the scar tissue every morning and evening in a firm up and down, vertical smoothing, stretching and softening motion to help any scar tissue remain soft and supple. We repeated this 'massage' six times every morning and every evening. I absolutely dreaded it but felt I was doing the best thing to make the frenulotomy a success. He was distressed whilst we performed the 'wound management' but calmed down very quickly once we'd finished (even without a feed). The tongue is still restricted, and I think it is a case of scar tissue rather than reattachment. Feeding didn't improve and I gave up breastfeeding, but he struggles with a bottle and I believe he needs a further division.

There are lots of anecdotal reports of the distress this type of intervention can cause. I have had several parents tell me they gave up doing it within a couple of days as they could not cope with seeing their baby in pain and distress. I have colleagues who have seen babies develop oral aversion and have episodes of bleeding, which can add to the distress. Infection is obviously also a concern. In 27 years of managing all kinds of wounds in my nursing roles, not once did I ever massage a healing wound to delay the healing process. Quite the contrary! Research and advice on wound healing tends to centre on leaving wounds undisturbed and minimising dressing changes as these can damage the delicate healing tissue.

There is no published research to support the safety or efficacy of disruptive wound massage after tongue-tie division. Furthermore, those promoting it do not agree on what type of disruption should be done. Should the wound be massaged vertically, horizontally or in a circle? Should the wound just be stretched and if so, in which plane? How often and for how long? There is no consensus. I have come across parents who have been told to massage the wound several times a day for eight weeks! Others have been told to just do it twice a day for just a few days.

I have also been contacted by mothers who have been asked to return repeatedly to practitioners to have the wound manually reopened to prevent recurrence. There is no evidence for any of this and parents need to be extremely cautious, in the absence of any published research, when following this type of aftercare and be made aware of the risks. Even if this type of intervention worked, the distress it can cause means it is not a satisfactory solution and many parents have told me they would rather go through a repeat division.

It is worth noting that some very well-known professionals in the field of lactation and tongue-tie have distanced themselves from strategies to disrupt the wound. Dr Jack Newman, a consultant paediatrician in Canada was an advocate, but in recent years has stopped recommending it as he does not feel it has any impact on outcomes.

Repeat division

It is difficult to find any accurate data on the numbers of repeat divisions being carried out and there are no specific research papers looking at the prevalence of tongue-tie recurrence and repeat divisions. Brookes and Bowley (2014) report a re-division rate of between 0.003–13%. It is a difficult issue to monitor as parents do not always re-present to professionals with ongoing feeding difficulties and will just manage it for themselves. If they do re-present it may not be to the original practitioner. In my local area many of the NHS services have age limits of 8–16 weeks, so I often see babies for assessment when recurrence is a concern as they have become too old to be reviewed by the NHS service. A recurrence can happen quite some time after the original division and it is not practical to follow up all babies for long periods. I have had babies return to me up to four months after division with recurrences. As it can take up to two years for wounds to remodel after healing we can perhaps expect recurrence at any point up to two years after division.

What is important is that babies are carefully assessed before considering a repeat division. In the past, when we had far less experience and understanding than we do now, far more repeat divisions were done. I have spoken to surgeons who have performed up to as many as seven divisions on a baby. But before doing a re-division we need to be clear that the feeding issues we are being presented with relate to a restriction in the tongue, are significant enough to warrant further surgery and cannot be resolved with conservative management. We also need to be able to differentiate between normal and abnormal healing.

I often have parents contacting me, sometimes within a couple of days of division, worrying that the tongue-tie has reattached because feeding is still difficult. We must be realistic. It takes time for babies to get used to the new range of movement in their tongues. It takes time for them to learn how to use their tongues to manage flow while co-ordinating the suck/swallow/breathe cycles. Some babies poke their tongues out beyond their lower lip immediately after division. Others do not. I have had babies who are feeding without any apparent issues brought back to me up to seven months after division due to concerns about them not sticking out their tongue, and will this affect their ability to lick an ice cream? All those babies have poked their tongues out at me when I have played with them and made liars of their parents, which of course is what children do! They always behave differently for others.

But why would some babies not immediately stick their tongues out? It could simply be that they don't realise they can because they couldn't do it prior to division. It could also be that there is some neck strain from birth and that this tension in the neck is causing some issues with the functioning of the nerve supply to the tongue, particularly the hypoglossal nerve, which controls movement of the intrinsic and extrinsic muscle of the tongue. Bodywork with an osteopath, chiropractor or cranial sacral therapist may help in this case along with lots of tummy time.

A conversation I had with the father of two babies I have

treated provided a further insight when he described his experience of division as a 12-year-old. He described his tongue after division as feeling like it wasn't attached to anything. He found poking it out very disconcerting as he had the overwhelming feeling it was going to drop out on to the floor, even though he knew it couldn't. Do babies feel like this? Is this why some don't poke their tongues out immediately? Probably not, because young babies do not have the intellectual capacity of a 12-year-old, but there is no doubt babies will notice the change in their tongue (they often seem to look a bit puzzled during the first feed post-division) and for some that may feel strange and unsettling. In the first few days there may also be some soreness, although adult reports of pain after division suggest this is mild in most cases.

However, muscle fatigue is not uncommon and again is something older children and adults report after division. This is where the tongue becomes tired, heavy and achy due to the muscles of the tongue being worked more and in a different way following release of the restriction. As one 13-year-old described it 'my tongue felt like a dead fish in the floor of my mouth'. Feeding is hard work with muscle fatigue, but it typically settles down within the first 10 days as the tongue tone improves. Lift of the tongue can also be affected by tongue tone and in cases where the frenulum has been very restrictive the tongue muscles are often weak and need time to strengthen before you will see the tongue lifting more. Tension in other muscles in the face and mouth (from the birthing process or from compensations used by the baby in the womb and after birth due to the restricted tongue) may also affect tongue lift. Some practitioners recommend facial and jaw massage to help release the muscles in the jaw, cheeks and lips.

Appearance of the wound post division can also be a worry for parents and professionals with limited knowledge of division. It is normal after the initial week or so of wound healing to be able to see a thin vertical strip of white tissue forming at the base of the tongue, as in the image below. This is a picture of a child whose tongue tie was divided as a baby due to very frequent feeding and slow weight gain and who successfully breastfed post-division, with better weight gain, into toddlerhood.

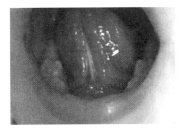

Normal healing in a 50% tongue-tie divided in the first few weeks of life a few years after division.

Some American practitioners talk about this strip of tissue being the 'new frenulum'. Most of us refer to it as normal scar tissue. Now, if this tissue becomes very thick and tight, impairs tongue function and affects feeding, then a conversation around re-division may follow. I am more inclined to consider re-division in cases where there was significant and sustained improvement after the first division before feeding deteriorated again. This is on the basis that if the first division didn't make a difference then we need to look again at other issues that could be impacting feeding, as re-dividing isn't likely to solve things. A lot of us who work with tongue-tied babies feel that muscular tensions and strains retained from birth may predispose a baby to the formation of tight scarring and ideally these tensions should be identified and addressed prior to the first division. However, they certainly need to be considered prior to any repeat division and I routinely suggest that all babies are assessed by an osteopath or chiropractor prior to a second division if they haven't already seen one.

Occasionally the cause of ongoing issues may be an incomplete divide. However, what is a complete divide? When I trained at Southampton (which before the retirement of Mervyn Griffiths was seen as the leading centre in the UK for tongue-tie division in babies and remains one of only two training centres in the country) I was taught to divide the frenulum until I could not feel any more tension under the tongue. Whether or not a diamond (or rhomboid)-shaped wound was achieved was not the focus. However, increasingly it was felt that you needed to achieve a diamond, exposing the genioglossus muscle, to achieve a full division and successful outcome. But achieving a diamond does not guarantee success. The idea that this is always necessary to achieve a good outcome came from conversations among practitioners in the USA without any research to back it up. The new studies on lingual frenulum anatomy mean that the idea of aiming for a deep, wide diamond as desirable is being questioned. With deep, wide wounds there may be more potential for damaging the lingual nerve. There is also concern about provoking a heavy bleed by cutting too deep and potentially damaging the muscle.

This concern can sometimes be a reason for doing an incomplete divide. Most experienced practitioners will have had cases where the anterior part of the tongue-tie is thin and divides well to expose a much tighter, thicker, more vascular looking posterior element, in some cases plastering the mouth floor close up to the under-surface of the tongue. We have to make a judgement about whether to proceed with further division, potentially risking a bleed or damaging other structures, such as the salivary glands, or leave the baby with an 'incomplete' division. In a community setting it is often safer to refer these cases for division by a surgeon in a hospital setting.

In practice many frenula divide to form a diamond and expose the genioglossus muscle because the tension in the frenulum pulls the mucous membrane and fascial layers apart as they are divided. But you may be able to get good outcomes with a relatively superficial division in some cases. Nikki Mills and colleagues (2019) report in their anatomy studies that cutting just the mucous membrane layer of the frenulum improved movement of the tongue.

Most experienced practitioners are cautious about performing re-divisions. We don't have any research on repeat divisions and outcomes. Repeat divisions have the potential to increase scarring, which can cause further tongue restriction and potentially make feeding worse.

Hannah, a mum of two children, who between them had five tongue-tie divisions, provides this sobering account:

My daughter, my first baby, did not latch to the breast for four days and was fed via syringe. We were then told to buy shields, she latched, and we went home. I knew absolutely nothing, only that I wanted to breastfeed. At 14 days old we were admitted to hospital for faltering growth after no one picking up on my concerns that she was sleeping for six hours, not pooing, not weeing, and had urates in her nappies. When we were admitted the infant feeding team midwife took one look in her mouth and said she had 100% tongue-tie and it was divided right there. At nine weeks old my HV noticed she clicked when feeding. We were advised to contact the infant feeding team again. They decided there was significant scar tissue, so a second division was done. [There were no other symptoms other than clicking and this did not resolve after division, but later did with good support with positioning and attachment]. At six months old, she would only sleep for short periods having previously slept all night. I didn't know anything about normal sleep behaviour and grandma suggested she must be suffering from wind. We saw a private practitioner who did a third division, advised that we apply stroking pressure to the wound and give her a dummy to stop further reattachment. [There was no improvement in sleep following this procedure and it is common for parents to report a sleep regression from 4–6 months of age which seems to be related to normal developmental changes.]

My son, when born gained weight very well but caused me significant pain and would be inconsolable every evening with 'colic'. We were referred and waited five weeks for an appointment. No one watched a feed but decided he needed a division, so it was done. Multiple exclusions to my diet saw some improvements but he was still so unhappy, so we had another assessment and the procedure was redone at 12 weeks. No one watched a feed. [There was pressure to do this second divide at this point due to the local NHS age limit.]

I am now studying to become an IBCLC having been a peer supporter for several years and I'm incredibly angry about my experiences. My daughter, no doubt at all, needed that first division, but I'm not convinced that any of the others were necessary. I honestly feel someone well qualified should have assessed us feeding because when I finally had some help from a IBCLC there were significant improvements to be made to positioning and attachment, this may have saved resources and time for everyone.

Bleeding

After recurrence of tongue-tie, bleeding is the most common complication we see and it is probably the thing that worries parents and practitioners the most. However, most babies will lose just a few drops to a teaspoon of blood, and in fact occasionally there is no bleeding at all. Because it is quite rare for a baby to bleed significantly after division there is little written about it. A report of two cases of prolonged and heavy bleeding requiring blood transfusion (Opara et al, 2012) highlighted the need for the procedure to be carried out by trained personnel. (These babies were treated by a traditional birth attendant and a community health worker.) A more recent paper on complications from New Zealand (Hale et al, 2019) reported on three cases of prolonged bleeding with one baby needing surgical intervention to stop the bleeding and a blood transfusion. This baby was identified as being vitamin K deficient despite having had vitamin K at birth, which is an unusual scenario.

Vitamin K deficiency is significant as vitamin K plays a role in blood clotting. All babies in the UK, and as far as I am aware in the developed world, are offered vitamin K prophylaxis at birth, either by one-off injection, or repeated doses of oral vitamin K. This is because babies are born with low levels of vitamin K, which predisposes newborns to bleeding into the gut or brain, and this can have serious consequences if not picked up and treated early enough. This condition is referred to as Vitamin K Deficiency Bleeding (VKDB), but was formerly known as haemorrhagic disease of the newborn. Exclusively breastfed babies are more at risk because breastmilk contains low levels of vitamin K (formula is fortified with vitamin K). Furthermore, we all rely on synthesis of vitamin K by the healthy bacteria in our gut, as well as on dietary sources. In babies these healthy bacteria take time to develop and of course can be disrupted by the administration of antibiotics to babies, which is not uncommon in early infancy. Birth interventions such as caesarean section can interfere with the healthy seeding of the baby's microbiome (gut bacteria). Babies who have not had vitamin K are more likely to have issues with clotting so there is a potential risk of more bleeding after a tongue-tie division. For this reason, practitioners performing division will ask whether the baby has had vitamin K, and some may refuse to do the division without it, or request the baby has a blood test to check their clotting first. Policies on this vary and, while babies can suffer a bleed due to vitamin K deficiency up to six months of age, the risk is less as the baby gets older so a risk assessment will take age into account, as well as whether the baby has had any formula or not.

The very first significant bleed I experienced was in a nine-day-old exclusively breastfed baby who was not transferring milk adequately and had not had the vitamin K injection. He bled for almost an hour and it did stop with pressure. When his clotting was checked he was found to be deficient in vitamin K and given the injection in the A&E department. It was fortunate that this was picked up as he may have gone on to have further internal bleeding. However, this has made me cautious in my practice and I think parents, while having a choice about whether or not to give their newborn vitamin K, do need to be accepting of the increased risk it may pose when it comes to division. The risk of a baby having any type of bleeding due to vitamin K deficiency is believed to be in the order of one in 11,000.

As well as being asked about whether your baby has had vitamin K or not, parents can also expect to be asked about bleeding disorders in the family. A bleeding disorder is a condition which prevents the blood from clotting and results in prolonged heavy bleeding. Bleeding disorders are often hereditary and the main ones we look for are haemophilia (type A and B), Von Willebrand's, Factor VII deficiency, Factor XI deficiency and platelet function disorders. If these conditions run in the family, there is a chance the baby could have them and so more detailed information will be needed. Advice may be sought from the Regional Haemophilia Centre on how to proceed and either the parents and/or the baby may need further tests to confirm or exclude a bleeding disorder prior to division.

Family medical history can be difficult to clarify and there can be misunderstandings within families and among professionals about how these conditions are inherited. This can be frustrating and upsetting for parents who just want to get on with 'fixing' the tongue-tie. But safety has to be paramount, as bleeding in the presence of these conditions can be hard to manage and of course it is unusual for newborns to exhibit signs. It is once they become mobile and start to knock and bruise themselves that a bleeding disorder often reveals itself.

However, there can be early warning signs of a problem such as a haematoma (blood-filled swelling) on the scalp, bleeding from the cord stump, significant bruising from the vitamin K injection or immunisations and prolonged bleeding after the heel-prick screening test, which is done on day 5–7 in the UK. All these things are worth mentioning when going for a tongue-tie division. Obviously liver or biliary disease and the use of anticoagulants (heparin) in babies will also increase the risk of bleeding and make division inadvisable, so a medical history of the baby should always be taken prior to division.

In terms of the incidence of bleeding we do have some information from an audit carried out by the Association of Tongue-tie Practitioners (ATP) in the UK in 2018 involving 50 practitioners who between them had carried out just under 77,000 procedures. There were 11 reported cases of babies requiring topical adrenaline applied to the wound to stop the bleeding and only one case where surgical intervention (in this case cautery) was needed. Most of the more prolonged and heavier bleeds will stop with pressure and that has been my experience.

The current ATP guidelines on the management of bleeding suggest applying pressure with damp gauze for 10 minutes initially and then a further 10 minutes. This can be uncomfortable for babies and 10 minutes seems like an awfully long time in this situation, but it does work well. The full guidelines can be accessed via the ATP website www.tongue-tie.org.uk and they are revised and updated regularly based on the experiences and feedback of members and any new research or treatments.

Within the ATP guidelines there is a section for parents because occasionally a baby will bleed at home. This can occur when the baby is moving their tongue around (which we obviously want to encourage) and inadvertently splits the wound open. Or the baby may catch the wound on a bottle teat, nipple shield, dummy or a finger they are sucking on. Older babies may poke the wound or catch it on a teething toy or similar. When this happens, bleeding is invariably light and will resolve spontaneously, with a short breast or bottle-feed, or a few minutes sucking on a dummy. However, a more significant bleed can occur so parents need to be given information about applying pressure and when to seek help. This is something your practitioner should explain to you, along with providing detailed information on the risk of bleeding and how it will be managed if it occurs immediately after division. This will enable you to make an informed decision about proceeding and ensures you know what to expect should it happen. This information can be scary to hear, but if your baby does bleed it will help allay some of the anxiety you will be feeling.

One mum I spoke to, whose baby suffered a prolonged bleed at home which necessitated transfer to hospital, told me how glad she was that the staff at the hospital where the division was carried out had prepared her and given her instructions on how long to feed baby for, how long to try pressure and at what point to seek hospital help. From her account I got a sense that this helped her stay calm, focused and in control.

Parents sometimes ask if there would be less bleeding with a laser division. The answer is not necessarily. Laser vapourises the tissue and the resultant heat cauterises the tissue in a similar way to electro cautery, which uses an electrical current to generate heat. However, this does not mean that there will be no bleeding at all, and it does not mean that the baby won't bleed once home as they will still be left with a wound. Some laser practitioners create more extensive wounds than those generally seen with scissors and they are more likely to recommend the disruptive wound management already discussed. Both factors may increase the risk of bleeding. Certainly, there have been cases of bleeding after laser division discussed on professional forums and by parents on social media. Dr Dermot Murnane, who provides laser division in Ireland, mentions bleeding after division on his website.

As well as recurrence and bleeding the NICE Guidance (2005) on *Division of Ankyloglossia (tongue-tie) for Breastfeeding* lists infection, ulceration, pain and damage to the tongue and submandibular ducts as other potential complications.

Infection

Infection is exceedingly rare. In 2010 there was a tragic case in the UK when a 17-day-old twin (Nicholas Baldwin) succumbed to *Klebsiella oxytoca* sepsis after a tongue-tie division. The coroner concluded that all the protocols had been followed and the infection was from an unknown source. *Klebsiella oxytoca* is carried in our guts and is considered a healthy bacterium. However, outside the gut it can cause serious infections. In most cases people make a good recovery unless they have weakened immunity. It is a bacterium commonly found in hospital and nursing home settings.

In breastfed babies milk passes directly from the breast to the baby so there is minimal risk of contamination and breastmilk contains antibodies which will help destroy any harmful bacteria that get into the wound. So infection of the wound is exceedingly rare in breastfed babies.

In babies who are completely formula-fed the risk is higher, as they will not be getting any antibodies and if bottles and teats are not thoroughly cleaned and sterilised there is a contamination risk. Furthermore, there is a significant risk if formula is not made up correctly. All formula should be prepared fresh at each feed and fed immediately and any that is left in the feeding bottle should be thrown away. Formula should not be prepared and stored in advance because it will quickly start to grow bacteria. Powdered formula needs to be prepared with very hot water at 70 degrees Celcius to kill off any bacteria within the powder because formula powder is not sterile and can be contaminated with bacteria during manufacture, before the can is sealed. The only way to ensure any bacteria are killed is to add it to water at 70 degrees. Bacteria in formula can cause gastroenteritis and more serious infections, as well as increasing the risk of a wound infection after division, so safe preparation is key. Some parents use formula preparation machines, but there are concerns about whether the shot of hot water added to the powder stays hot long enough to kill off the bacteria. Using ready-made formula while the wound heals is the safest option if you are formula-feeding, but this is expensive. The only wound infection I have seen in a baby I treated occurred a week after division. The parents had been putting boiled water in the fridge and storing it and then adding the powder to this cold water and warming it up, so I have no doubt that this was the source of the bacteria.

Ulceration is not something I have ever come across. The wound forms a white scab, which looks like a mouth ulcer, after division and this scab gradually shrinks and disappears over a period of 7–14 days as the wound heals. I wonder if this is what NICE is referring to. The scab can have a slight yellow or greenish tinge to it and will look very yellow/orange in a baby with jaundice. But this is normal healing. In the case of an infection the wound may look red and inflamed round the edges and be weepy. The baby may also develop a temperature.

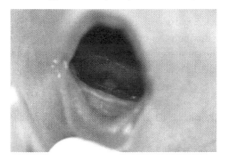

Normal wound healing two days after division

Occasionally the wound over-granulates as it heals, creating a ridge or flap of proud flesh under the tongue, which one mum described to me as looking like 'a small extra tongue'. This usually happens within the first two weeks of healing and resolves as the wound remodels in the first 2–3 months. It does not seem to bother the baby in the cases I have seen. Over-granulation can happen in any open wound as it heals, not just following tongue-tie division.

Pain

Pain in babies can be difficult to assess but there is no doubt that babies feel pain when undergoing procedures. Research using MRI scans of the brain has confirmed this. Furthermore, we now know, with the publication of the research in 2019 on frenulum anatomy (Mills et al, 2019) that branches of the lingual nerve do extend into the lingual frenulum. It was previously thought the lingual frenulum was poorly innervated and lacked sensation. That said, most babies tolerate the procedure well. Reports from adults who have had division without any anaesthetic (such as the well-known Dr Alison Hazelbaker) suggest that there is only a mild stinging sensation during scissor division and the wound is not too sore unless you poke at it. However babies, like adults, are individuals and will experience pain and discomfort differently. I have had babies sleep through the procedure and this has been reported in some of the published studies too (Hogan et al, 2005). But I have also had some that have been quite upset both during and after the procedure. Whether the upset related to them being hungry, being swaddled and held still or feeling some pain during the procedure is difficult to judge. Any upset is likely to be due to a combination of factors. Usually any crying is short-lived. In a case series of 215 babies with an average age of 19 days by Mervyn Griffiths (2004), 99% of the babies cried for less than a minute after division, with 85% crying for less than 20 seconds. We use breastfeeding immediately after division whenever we can as this is known to have analgesic effects, as reported in a Cochrane Systematic Review (Shah et al, 2012):

> Breastfeeding provides pain relief for newborn babies undergoing painful procedures. Medicine for pain relief is commonly given for major painful procedures but may not be given for minor painful procedures such as blood

sampling (by heel-prick or venepuncture). There are different forms of non-pharmacological strategies that may be used to reduce pain in babies, such as holding, swaddling them, sucking on a pacifier, or giving sweet solutions (such as sucrose or glucose). Different studies done in babies have shown that breastfeeding is a good way to reduce the pain babies feel when subjected to minor painful procedures. These studies have been done in full-term babies and they have shown that breastfeeding is effective by demonstrating that it reduces babies' crying time and reduces different pain scores that have been validated for babies. Breastmilk given by syringe has not shown the same efficacy as breastfeeding itself.

Breastfeeding immediately before division can also have a calming effect, which tends to reduce crying during the procedure and afterwards in my experience. Taking a swab soaked in mum's breastmilk and wiping this around baby's mouth pre and post-division is another option. Where breastfeeding or breastmilk are not options sucrose solution is sometimes used before and after division.

Just the smell of breastmilk can be calming and have a pain-relieving effect according to a study of 84 babies by Tasci et al (2020). Filter papers soaked in either breastmilk or formula, according to the baby's usual feeding method, were held under the baby's nose for three minutes during the heel-prick test on day five after birth. Response was measured through crying, cortisol levels in saliva samples, the Neonatal Infant Pain Score and monitoring of heart rate and oxygen levels. The results demonstrated that: 'The pain threshold and heart rates of the newborn in the breastmilk group were significantly lower than those in the formula milk group ($p < 0.001$). Salivary cortisol in the formula milk group increased and oxygen saturation levels in these infants decreased significantly more as compared to the breastmilk group ($p < 0.05$).' The authors concluded that the odour of breastmilk may be helpful in reducing pain during heel-prick blood sampling, and it seems reasonable to suppose a similar effect could be seen with tongue-tie division. So keeping mum in close proximity to baby during the procedure and not removing baby to another room, or having a pad soaked in breastmilk close to the baby, may be soothing.

For babies who are not breastfed, a bottle-feed or pacifier (dummy), with or without sucrose, can be offered to soothe them. For all babies over 12 weeks old I suggest parents give a dose of infant paracetamol before the division. Babies over eight weeks old can have a dose of infant paracetamol after the division should they appear in pain, but very few parents report this is necessary.

When I did my training in division in Southampton in 2011, Carolyn Westcott told me that they had done a short trial using local anaesthetic gel on the frenulum prior to division to see if this reduced crying and distress. Apparently, the babies did not like the taste of the gel and after division found it harder to feed due to the numbness caused by the gel. Duration of crying and bleeding increased so they did not continue with this practice.

We should expect babies to be unsettled and cry more than usual in the first 24 hours after division and be fussy with feeding while they get used to the new movement in their tongue. As well as the wound being a bit sore, they may also suffer to some extent with muscle fatigue. The tongue muscle in a baby with a tongue-tie will not have developed properly due to the restriction in movement so once the baby moves it more then they may very well experience some aching and heaviness in that muscle. Breastfeeding is the primary strategy for soothing babies through this period, but obviously this may not be easy. Fortunately, skin-to-skin is another strategy which can be used with all babies and a Cochrane systematic review on Kangaroo care (which keeps premature and sick babies in skin-to-skin with a parent or caregiver during hospitalisation) concluded that skin-to-skin seems to reduce the pain response to procedures and speeds up recovery.

Some authorities claim that using laser for tongue-tie division results in reduced pain. However, Effath Yasmin (an IBCLC in India), during an online conference presentation in 2019 for GOLD Learning Online Continuing Education, reported that in a small survey of seven practitioners, those using laser reported significantly more need for post-division pain relief in the first 24–72 hours than those using scissors or scalpels. This may be due to delayed healing and inadvertent laser-induced thermal injury (Devishree et al, 2012).

Breast refusal

Occasionally babies will completely refuse the breast after division and this seems to happen more in younger babies who are not well established on the breast (typically those that are less than ten days old) and have extensive tongue-ties where tongue tone is poor afterwards. Lots of skin-to-skin, finger-feeding to develop tongue tone and placement and sometimes nipple shields can be useful in getting baby back to the breast, and the rejection of the breast usually resolves within a few days. I have also occasionally seen this in older babies, often where milk supply is compromised and they have had regular exposure to bottles. They then reject the breast in favour of the 'easier' flow of the bottle. Babies with a long history of unresolved reflux may also reject the breast as they may already have a degree of aversion and negative association with the breast if the reflux has caused pain and distress.

Damage to the tongue and submandibular ducts.

There is always a risk of damage to other structures when doing a division because we are using scissors in a small cavity and the oral structures are in close proximity to each other. But surprisingly damage to other structures is exceedingly rare, and in most cases will heal. As a practitioner I am mindful of the potential to damage the submandibular ducts (the salivary tissue/glands), especially when dividing anterior frenula that are short and tight, where the salivary tissue bisects the frenulum. Damage to the submandibular ducts can result in the formation of a ranula (a type of cyst) which may very well resolve on its own but could require surgical repair. This type of complication seems, anecdotally, to be more common in the USA where they do more laser divisions and wounds can be more extensive. I have seen one baby, who was treated by a colleague, develop a swelling in the floor of the mouth after division which was attributed to submandibular duct damage. This swelling did not seem to bother the baby and resolved spontaneously after a number of weeks. If I am in any doubt about potential damage, I will refer the baby to a surgeon for division and I know many of my midwifery and nursing colleagues do the same.

Damage to the lingual nerve

Concerns have been raised about the potential for lingual nerve damage by Nikki Mills and her fellow researchers following their studies on the anatomy of the lingual frenulum, particularly in relation to laser division, or where the wound created is wide or deep:

Our study has shown these nerve branches to be located superficially on the ventral tongue surface, immediately beneath the fascia, placing them at risk for direct or transmitted thermal injury during frenotomy. Risk of temporary or permanent neural injury would be higher when: the incision is deep (any incision that cuts into genioglossus), frenotomy performed with any tool that utilizes thermal energy (which is absorbed into underlying tissues), and/or any procedure where the incision extends widely from the midline. (Mills et al, 2019)

Injuries to nerves can result in changes in sensation (pain or numbness). In most cases it is believed these changes will be temporary, but there is a lack of research in relation to tongue-tie division and lingual nerve damage in both infant and older child and adult populations.

Despite these risks the NICE Guidance (2005) states:

Current evidence suggests that there are no major safety concerns about division of ankyloglossia (tongue-tie) and limited evidence suggests that this procedure can improve breastfeeding. This evidence is adequate to support the use of the procedure provided that normal arrangements are in place for consent, audit, and clinical governance.

The NICE position on this has not changed and none of the five randomised control trials on frenulotomy in infants included in a Cochrane review reported any adverse outcomes (O'Shea et al, 2017).

Effectiveness of treatment

As a parent, if you are going to put your baby through a surgical procedure, which is not without risk, you need some assurance that it will help improve the feeding difficulties you are experiencing. Obviously robust assessment, as we have seen, is essential in ensuring that this procedure is used appropriately and only offered to those babies who will benefit from it.

But what do the studies on tongue-tie tell us about efficacy? Most of the studies to date have focused on nipple pain, although some have also included measures looking at weight gain and milk transfer. There is one study that has looked specifically at reflux. There is little research on outcomes in bottle-fed babies, with the focus being on those that are breastfed. However, seven out of eight systematic reviews have concluded that while the quality of the evidence may be weak to moderate, in most studies there was evidence of improvements in feeding. In the appendix you can find a summary of some of the better known studies.

A survey conducted in New Zealand by Illing et al (2019) of 176 parents of infants aged under six months, who had had division (in a clinic run by a GP and IBCLC) found that 98% of these parents would seek division again in similar circumstances. In practice I certainly see lots of babies for division whose older siblings had the procedure and these parents are usually very keen to proceed, reporting positive outcomes previously. This survey also found that reported breastfeeding times and nipple pain scores were reduced at follow-up at around 23 days post-division. At the time of division 93 babies were not fully breastfeeding but following the procedure 33 of these were able to establish full breastfeeding. Eleven mothers reported a decline in breastfeeding post-division, with two moving from full breastfeeding to full formula-feeding and the other nine moving from partial breastfeeding (combination feeding) to full formula-feeding. One baby had to be syringe-fed for two weeks following division and then re-established breastfeeding. I have seen this happen in cases where the tongue is severely restricted and as a result tongue tone has been poor afterwards. It is also a risk in situations of very low supply. I also had a case where the baby refused to latch after division due to significant jaw tension which resolved with osteopathic input. This baby went on to breastfeed for over three years. Three babies experienced reattachment of the frenulum.

Many studies have been criticised because of their small sample size, their methodology (several have no control group and only recorded short-term outcomes) and the lack of long-term follow-up. Ethically it is difficult to withhold an intervention which appears to be beneficial. In the published studies that did have a control group, most of the control group were offered division shortly after it became clear that there were improvements being seen in the intervention groups. Thus the controls were lost, making long-term comparisons impossible. There are also difficulties in attributing long-term outcomes to the procedure because there are so many factors which influence successful breastfeeding outcomes. Delays in diagnosis and treatment of tongue-tie may result in loss of confidence in the mother, poor weight gain, low milk supply and supplementation with formula, which will all shorten the duration of breastfeeding. Furthermore, access to skilled ongoing breastfeeding support is not universally available and healthcare workers' education in infant feeding is inconsistent. Social pressures in terms of family support, the need to return to work, how breastfeeding is portrayed in the media and so on will all influence how long a mother breastfeeds for too. So, outcomes are not simply going to be related to whether frenulotomy was a success or not.

There is a study being conducted currently by NPEU, Oxford University which is a multi-centred randomised trial for 'babies with breastfeeding difficulties who are thought to have tongue-tie and who are receiving breastfeeding support and there is uncertainty about whether frenotomy would help continuation of breastfeeding. The aim of the trial is to find out if skilled support for breastfeeding on its own, or together with a frenotomy helps mothers and their babies to breastfeed'. (www.npeu.ox.ac.uk/frosttie). However, this study was due to be completed by 2021 and has been delayed by the pandemic. While some commentators are saying it will provide definitive evidence on whether division is effective or not I am not sure the scope and design of the study has the power to do this. However, it will certainly add to the evidence base and that must be a good thing.

Whatever the limitations and controversies within the available research, one thing we must never forget are the experiences of parents on this issue. The following experiences were shared on my Facebook page:

Success stories

I had no success getting my daughter to latch on in hospital – she just struggled with it, despite the midwives trying their best. I was told fairly early on that she didn't have a tongue-tie, so I assumed it was my incompetence... you can imagine how that felt! We were only allowed to leave hospital when we told them we'd bottle/syringe-feed and that we had bought a pump. I pumped (almost 24/7... I was exhausted) while husband syringe-fed her small amounts round the clock. I was so desperate to breastfeed her, and came to one of the Ely Milks clinics when she was about 10 days old. She was immediately diagnosed with a posterior TT, and we arranged to have it cut by you, which you did when she was three weeks old. After a fair amount of screaming, she latched on and fed for about an hour (first time she'd done that!). However, a couple of days after that, she started refusing to latch on (I think you'd warned us that this might happen, but to keep trying/offering). Eventually, she finally got the hang of it at six weeks old, and never looked back! She finally stopped nursing at 3.5 years (my choice), even continuing while I was pregnant with her little brother (I fed both of them for about six months). She kept feeding – even when she was nil-by-mouth following major abdominal surgery at six months (I expressed and she just picked up after).

My twin boy had a thick posterior tie. I had severe damage to my nipple, it looked like it had a crater in the middle due to his suck. My GP was dismissive, the receptionist got an earful as she suggested if he would take a bottle they wouldn't touch it. The local ENT wouldn't do it properly and sent me a letter telling me my problem was feeding twins. I saw an IBCLC and tongue-tie practitioner who referred me on and helped me get to the right private practitioner to have it revised as it was too thick to be done in the community setting in case of a large bleed. The feed immediately after the revision, at four months of age, was immediately 100% gentler and I have just fed him to sleep for his nap at two years of age. The revision 100% saved our breastfeeding journey.

We had the tongue-tie done when our daughter was three months old, and by this point was bottle-fed, we had screaming bouts after every feed, we even explored CMPA [Cows Milk Protein Allergy] *with the doctor, change of formula/bottles, reflux, colic, it got to the point we didn't want to feed her in public because of her reaction. Once the tongue-tie was done, it was like we had a different baby, almost instantly. She was settled and content and feeding peacefully. It made a huge difference to our life.*

We had struggled with feeding for the first three weeks of her life. Following tie division she fed straight away with no problem latching. That night she slept for six hours and was genuinely content. We had been coerced into bottle-feeding in the early days, owing to latching problems. We were extremely lucky that she would take freely from either the bottle or the breast!

My third baby had a posterior tongue-tie snipped at around six weeks old. I breastfed my first two into toddlerhood and am trained in breastfeeding myself, but I had bleeding nipples in week one and he was so unhappy with wind and reflux. We managed to improve things with positioning but I was still in pain when feeding. After the snip breastfeeding was immediately more comfortable and he is now able to maintain his latch so much better. He is still windy and refluxy but much less, and he is generally much more cheerful as well.

Feeding dramatically improved for us. From the first feed after division I didn't need a nipple shield anymore (after needing one every feed for the whole first three weeks of his life) he went from feeding for 1–2 minutes every 15–20 minutes to feeding fully for 20ish minutes every 3–4 hours. My nipples healed up finally and we continued to feed until he was two.

Some stories with less successful outcomes

Child three had a small posterior tongue-tie that caused her to feed constantly. Left me in great pain and she was a very unhappy unsettled baby. She lost 8% on day five and I had mastitis on day six. Her tongue-tie was snipped on day nine although was nearly declined as so small. She lost weight again on day 14 dropping to 11%

of her weight despite the fact feeding was pain-free. She continued to be very hard to feed, unable to maintain suction and struggling. Top-ups were given to help with the weight as a mix of expressed breastmilk and formula. Saw an IBCLC who suggested CMPA as she had green nappies, severe rashes and was miserable. Baby gained weight and we did discover she had CMPA. At six weeks her tongue was checked and felt to still be restricted. At 14 weeks she was seen and had it re-cut. Didn't bring a great deal of difference to feeding. By six months baby was diagnosed with multiple allergies and finally around month seven she started to settle and be happy.

Second baby (lockdown) tongue-tie divided at eight weeks, hoped it would make a difference but still had bleeding nipples, aching boobs and mastitis symptoms every three days so had to stop feeding at three months. I think my boobs felt worse after the division. I still think I just had too much supply which never settled and poor latch. Baby was settled and putting on weight fine.

Are there any babies who shouldn't be treated?

The Australian Dental Association, in its *Ankyloglossia and Oral Frena Consensus Statement* (2020), lists the following as contraindications to division: orofacial malformations such as cleft palate, Pierre Robin Sequence, bleeding disorders, neuromuscular conditions and vitamin K deficiency.

We have already discussed bleeding disorder and vitamin K deficiency. Babies with liver or biliary disease may also be more prone to bleeding, as would babies on anticoagulant therapy, so this would make division inadvisable.

Pierre Robin Sequence is a condition which is present at

birth. The baby will have a smaller than normal lower jaw, a tongue that is placed further back than normal and an opening in the roof of the mouth (cleft palate). Babies with this condition will have difficulties with breathing and feeding and releasing any tongue-tie can cause airway obstruction, so it is an absolute contraindication.

Neuromuscular conditions such as Down's syndrome, particularly where low muscle tone is a feature, also require careful assessment by the multidisciplinary team caring for the child before any decision about the appropriateness of division is made.

Caution also needs to be exercised in babies who have been diagnosed with a 'floppy larynx' (laryngomalacia) which again is a condition of low tone, this time of the larynx. This is a relatively common diagnosis, and in these situations I will seek guidance from the ENT consultant caring for the baby in relation to the laryngomalacia.

Congenital heart conditions do not prohibit division. However, consideration needs to be given to how compromised the baby is as a result of the heart condition and how they would cope in the event of a bleed. These babies are generally treated in a hospital environment, except in the case of babies with milder heart murmurs (ventricular septal defects).

So, if your baby has a pre-existing health problem or is on medication it is important to ensure the practitioner offering division is fully aware of this. Do expect them to consult with the medical team caring for your baby before going ahead with a procedure. This can be frustrating as it will cause delay, but safety and the best interests of your baby are paramount.

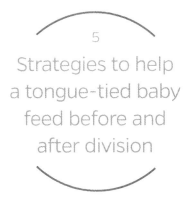

5

Strategies to help a tongue-tied baby feed before and after division

Not all babies with a tongue-tie will need a division and not all parents will choose for their baby to have a division. Those babies that do have a division will need support with feeding both before and after division.

The priority is always to feed the baby. Some babies with a tongue-tie, as we have already discussed, will be unable to latch to the breast at all. Some will latch but will struggle to sustain the latch and will repeatedly break the seal or slip off or down the nipple. Some babies will struggle to create sufficient vacuum to transfer milk effectively. In the early days these babies are at risk of developing low blood sugars, jaundice, dehydration, high sodium levels and above average weight loss and may continue to struggle to get sufficient nutrition to maintain energy levels and grow. This situation can then become a vicious circle as a lack of milk intake reduces the passage of meconium through the bowel, leading to a rise in bilirubin levels and jaundice. The jaundice, along with a low-calorie intake and associated reduced energy levels, then impacts on feeding at the breast with the baby tiring more quickly. So feeds become shorter and potentially less frequent. The whole situation can be tiring and demoralising for both mum and baby and left unchecked can endanger the health of the baby.

In an ideal world all newborn babies would be observed feeding in the first few hours after birth by someone skilled in breastfeeding assessment and support to ensure that the baby is achieving an effective and comfortable latch, and is adequately transferring milk. Parents would be coached in how to position baby at the breast and what to look out for to ensure their baby is feeding effectively and getting enough milk. However, with staffing shortages, limited training in infant feeding and pressure for early discharge this often doesn't happen, and parents can arrive home full of uncertainty about what to expect and anxiety about getting things right.

So as a parent of a newborn – not just a newborn with a tongue-tie, as many tongue-ties are not identified until several weeks or even months after birth – what do you need to know?

How to latch your baby to the breast

Firstly, it is helpful to know how to position your baby at the breast. The acronym CHINS is often used to help parents remember the key principles:

> C – close
> H – head free
> I – in line
> N – nose to nipple
> S – sustainable

Your baby needs to be held tucked in close to your body, so you are touching each other. They need to be able to tilt their head back, so any support needs to be given around the shoulders and neck. There should be no touching of your baby's head and forcing them to the breast. Your baby's body and head need to be in alignment facing the breast, so the neck and spine are straight and not twisted. We do not drink with our heads turned to one side as it is uncomfortable and makes swallowing more difficult and the same holds true for babies. Your baby needs to be lined up so their nose, and not their mouth, is opposite the nipple. This encourages them to tilt their head back as they reach up for the nipple and helps to ensure an asymmetric latch, with the nipple positioned up into the roof of the mouth and the nipple tip reaching the junction of the hard and soft palate. This is essential for a comfortable latch. Finally, once latched on the position you and your baby find yourselves in needs to be sustainable, so you need your back supported, your shoulders relaxed. The weight of your baby needs to be well supported, either by your body or arms or with the addition of a small pillow, cushion or rolled/folded blanket or towel under your baby or under your arm, once baby has latched. Nursing pillows are often too bulky and place your baby in a position which is 'too high' to attach well to the breast and are generally best avoided. However, for babies who are struggling to sustain the latch and keep slipping off, where you have a wrist injury, or for twins they can be useful in helping to 'wedge' the baby in place at the breast.

There are a variety of positions that can be used for breastfeeding. One of the most helpful for babies who are struggling to latch, who have perhaps been 'manhandled' at the breast, or who are causing pain and damage to the nipples, is the 'laid-back' position. In this position you adopt a semi-recumbent position and lie your baby on their tummy either vertically or diagonally across your chest so their mouth is positioned very close to the nipple and they can use their hands, chin, lips and tongue to explore and find the nipple and self-attach. Babies relax when in skin-to-skin and when on their tummies so this position tends to have a calming effect and they will often be more patient and persistent in their attempts to latch. Once attached, the lower jaw will be more relaxed leading to a reduction in 'biting' and 'clamping' behaviours which can cause nipple pain and trauma.

However, not all babies with a tongue-tie have sufficient tongue extension to allow them to scoop up the breast and latch in these laid-back positions. Side-lying is an alternative where both you and your baby lie on your sides facing each other and your baby is then tucked in close with their tummy tucked up against your tummy so their head naturally tilts back, with their nose opposite the nipple, ready for latching. The cradle hold, cross-cradle hold, underarm (sometimes called the rugby ball hold) and the upright saddle hold (also known as the koala hold) are also options. See this link for information on positions: www.llli.org/breastfeeding-info/positioning.

In practice I find a lot of the parents who come to me are using the cross-cradle hold or underarm hold. This is probably because these are commonly taught, and for babies who are tongue-tied and struggling to latch they can enable parents to assist the baby in latching and staying latched, perhaps more so than some of the other positions. In these positions, and the saddle hold, it is possible to use specific latching techniques which may be particularly helpful in babies who are tongue-tied. These techniques are the exaggerated latch (also known as the 'flipple' or 'nipple flick') and breast shaping.

The exaggerated latch
With this technique your baby is placed at the breast in the cross-cradle, underarm or saddle hold with their nose opposite the nipple. You then 'exaggerate' this nose to nipple

position by using your thumb or finger to tilt the nipple upwards. When your baby tilts their head back, opens wide and comes on to the breast, you 'flick' the nipple under the top lip to help get the tip of the nipple deep into the mouth to the junction of the hard/soft palate, fill the roof of the mouth with breast tissue and get as much breast tissue in over the lower lip as possible to achieve a deep, comfortable, secure and effective latch. This can be particularly effective for tongue-tied babies as the deeper latch helps to secure the breast in the mouth and reduces slipping and loss of suction (clicking). It can also help to fill the extra space created by a high palate, so often seen in association with a tongue-tie as we have discussed, and this can reduce nipple pain and pinching.

Breast shaping

Breast shaping is a useful technique for mums with flatter nipples or larger and fuller breasts. It is particularly useful for babies with tongue-tie as flat nipples are an added challenge for them as they do not have the tongue extension to help locate the nipple and draw the breast in easily. Shaping the breast makes the nipple area more prominent for the baby. Babies with tongue-tie also often struggle to achieve a wide gape due to tension in the lower jaw from the tongue-tie. Breast shaping effectively narrows or squashes the area they are trying to latch on to, which makes attaching to the breast easier. It can be helpful to think of the breast as being a bit like a thick hamburger. We need to make it flatter to fit it into our mouth. Breast shaping also helps to take the weight of a large breast off the baby's chin, lower jaw, and chest and this may help the baby to latch and feed more easily with deeper jaw movement.

The breast can be shaped by placing the hand on the same side as the breast, either underneath the breast with the thumb on the outer aspect and fingers on the inner side making a 'U' shape, or by placing the thumb on top of the breast in the 12 o'clock position and the fingers underneath the breast in the 6 o'clock position to form a 'C' shape. The 'U' shape is used for cradle positions and the 'C' shape for saddle and underarm holds. Once the baby has latched and feels secure at the breast the hand can be carefully removed.

Breast shaping can be combined with the exaggerated latch using the thumb to tilt the nipple up and flick it under the bottom lip.

> *Justine* (LLL Leader) *helped me to get a comfortable latch when I was struggling with uncomfortable feeding with my second baby. She showed me how to try the koala hold with flipple which really helped, making sure baby was really close tummy to tummy and below my breast so he had to look up, getting that nice big gape. The discomfort I was feeling in other positions disappeared when I tried this for the first time.* Catriona

> *Laid-back breastfeeding, with my thumb above the areola (where baby's nose is) to flip the nipple past the hard palate helped me. Also looking at my breast (no bra on) so I could see how they hung and the direction of my nipples really helped too. Laid-back worked better on my right breast and cradle worked better on my left, with my right boob flopped over baby's body.* Asha

How do I know if the latch is effective?

It is important that parents know how to check that their baby is latched on to the breast effectively. Things to look for are:

- The baby has a large mouthful of breast and their mouth is wide open.

- The baby's chin is touching the breast with their nose tilted slightly away from the breast so they can breathe.
- The latch is asymmetric, meaning you can see more areola (the skin around the nipple) above the baby's top lip than below the lower lip. (In very pale skin or if your areola is small this may be difficult to see.)
- Feeding is comfortable.
- There should be no change in the shape or colour of the nipple after feeding. The nipple should not look pinched, ridged or white after feeds.
- Baby's cheeks are rounded during sucking with no dimpling.
- When baby first latches sucks will be shallow and frequent to stimulate the let-down. Once the milk is flowing the rhythm changes to slower, deeper sucks with swallowing you can see or hear. There will be short pauses from time to time and the suck to swallow ratio should be no more than three sucks per swallow.
- At the end of the feed the baby comes off on their own and is calm and satisfied.

Your baby should also produce plenty of wet and dirty nappies. As a guide we look for at least 1–2 heavy wet nappies in 24 hours in the first two days and 1–2 stools, which will be black. By day three we would expect at least three heavy wet nappies and two stools which are turning green/brown, and from day four at least four heavy wet nappies and two brown/yellow stools. By day five it's at least five wet nappies and two yellow stools and from day six onwards at least six heavy wet nappies and two yellow stools in 24 hours. Stools should be at least the size of a £2 coin. From six weeks stool output slows and it is not uncommon for babies to miss a few days between stools at this stage, but we would always expect at least six heavy wet nappies.

What about babies who will not latch?

When a baby cannot latch due to tongue-tie, or struggles to latch initially after division, this can be a huge challenge on a practical level, because how are you going to feed this baby? It can also be emotionally tough and feel like a rejection by the baby. However, babies instinctively want to feed. For all babies feeding is about survival. They aren't lazy or choosing not to latch. If latching is a struggle there will be a reason. That reason is often a physical one.

A tongue-tie can obviously make latching to the breast extremely difficult and for some babies impossible due to the restriction in tongue extension. But other factors such as birth interventions, including forceps and ventouse, can leave babies feeling sore, and in some cases physically bruised and damaged, which can make breastfeeding uncomfortable for them. Suctioning to clear the airway after birth or investigations and examinations which involve going into the mouth can set up an oral aversion. 'Manhandling' at the breast by well-intentioned midwives can also set up a breast aversion. But what can be done about this?

Skin-to-skin is the place to start. It calms your baby and reduces stress by stabilising breathing, heart rate, temperature, and blood sugars. It allows your baby to explore the breast in their own time and attempt to latch when they are ready. It also calms you and triggers the release of the hormone prolactin, which drives milk production, and oxytocin, which is the hormone that triggers the 'let-down' of milk by causing the smooth muscle in the alveoli (milk sacs) to contract. Colostrum or milk may then start to leak from your breast, which can encourage your baby to latch. Patience and persistence are needed as it may take your baby several attempts before they are successful.

'Rebirthing' is another strategy which can enhance the

effects of skin-to-skin by recreating the birth environment to help trigger the newborn reflexes that help a baby to initiate feeding. To do this run a deep bath of warm water at a temperature safe and comfortable for your baby, which is likely to be cooler than your usual bath water temperature. You should then get into the bath and have a partner or helper pass your baby to you. Your baby is then placed on your chest (both of you being naked) and given the opportunity to explore the breast. You can both be kept warm by your partner or helper pouring warm water gently over you both.

Another strategy to try is latching in motion. Latching while standing and rocking baby, or while sitting on a birth ball and bouncing, can calm a baby who is fractious at the breast and struggling to latch.

If these methods fail, then a nipple shield can be a game-changer in terms of getting your baby to latch. Lots of babies seem to be able to get the hang of latching with a shield as the firm silicone provides more sensory stimulation. However, it is vital that the shield is the right size for both the nipple and the baby, as a shield that doesn't fit correctly can make it difficult for your baby to remove milk from the breast and lead to nipple trauma. As well as varying sizes of shields being available, they also come in different shapes, some being more bulbous and others being more tapered. The thickness and texture of the silicone can also vary between brands, with some being thinner and more flexible than others. Advice should be sought, ideally from an IBCLC or someone equally skilled in breastfeeding, to ensure the correct fit and that the baby is able to remove milk from the breast with a shield. This is particularly important in babies with a tongue-tie as they often have difficulty creating sufficient vacuum to draw the milk from the breast due to the restriction in tongue elevation. A shield can create a further barrier to milk flow and mean that some tongue-tied babies simply cannot draw milk through the shield at all or their intake at the breast is compromised. I have seen weight plummet after a shield was used without checking whether the baby was able to draw milk through the shield effectively. Some mothers will also find that nipple pain increases with the use of a shield due to the baby employing compensatory strategies to draw milk from the breast.

A further issue with shields is that once a baby has started using them it can take some time to wean off them. However, with all that said shields do have a place and can be an effective way of establishing breastfeeding in a baby who can otherwise not latch. Most mothers prefer to be able to breastfeed with a shield, than to have to express 8–10 times in 24 hours for a non-latching baby!

Feeding the non-latching baby or the baby who is not getting enough milk

The first rule of lactation practice is to feed the baby. The second is to protect the milk supply. Expressing milk fulfils both these functions.

If a baby doesn't latch after birth, expressing needs to start as soon as possible and certainly within six hours of birth. The frequent stimulation and drainage of the breast will not only provide colostrum for feeding the baby, but will also stimulate the further development of the breast tissue, activate the prolactin receptors, and ensure supply is established and maintained into the future. All too often when a baby isn't latching or isn't latching well and is unsettled due to hunger, losing weight or causing nipple pain and damage, formula is introduced without any suggestion that mum could express, and without any information being given on why this is important or the long-term impact of formula supplementation on milk supply.

No one enjoys expressing, but the sooner it is implemented

and the more frequently it is done the easier it will be to resolve the feeding issues once the tongue-tie is divided, or to sustain at least some breastfeeding if the tongue-tie isn't going to be divided for any reason. A newborn baby will happily suckle on an empty or near-empty breast. But the first ten weeks is when most brain development occurs, and it does not take many weeks for babies to become much more aware of flow at the breast and need an incentive to stay latched on. For example, a four-week-old baby who has been predominantly formula-fed due to early excessive weight loss at day three, whose mother has only been expressing once or twice a day since, is not likely to latch and stay at the breast more than briefly, even after tongue-tie division. These brief feedings alone are not likely to be sufficient to repair a compromised milk supply. Milk supply is arguably the most important factor in resolving breastfeeding difficulties, alongside the determination of the mother and the support around her.

So how often does a mother need to express? That will depend on her situation. If baby is not going on the breast at all, or cannot remove milk from the breast, then expressing needs to occur eight to ten times per day (24-hour period), both breasts for 10–20 minutes, to mimic a baby's normal frequency. The hormone prolactin, which stimulates milk production, peaks overnight so at least one expressing session during the night is recommended to optimise supply. In cases where a baby is latching and getting some milk, but not enough to gain adequate weight, then expressing both breasts one to four times in 24 hours to provide the milk needed for top-ups and to boost supply may be adequate. It depends on how slow the weight gain is. (A gain of around 25–30g per day is considered adequate in the first three months of life.)

Hand expressing in the first few days, before the milk comes in, is much more effective than using a pump as colostrum is only produced in small amounts. You should not expect to get more than half a teaspoon (a couple of millilitres) out at a time. However, amounts vary considerably from mother to mother and time and practice will increase the amounts expressed. Once the milk comes in at around day 3–5 then a pump can be used. If a mum needs to pump more than about three times per day then a double electric pump will be the most efficient as both breasts can be expressed at the same time, reducing the time spent by half. Double pumping also seems to be more effective in increasing supply. A study by Hill et al (1996) found that prolactin levels were higher in mums of preterm babies who expressed both breasts simultaneously compared to those who expressed one breast after the other.

For mothers needing to express less often a single electric pump or a manual pump may be adequate. There is a huge variety of breast pumps available. Techniques such as 'hands-on pumping', which uses compression by hand to increase breast drainage while pumping (Morton et al 2009), and 'power pumping', which mimics the cluster-feeding newborns tend to do, especially in the evenings, can help increase supply and the amounts expressed. An IBCLC or someone with equivalent training and skills can help you to choose the right breast pump, and develop an expressing plan and techniques to suit your situation. It is always important to keep in mind that while the tongue-tie may be the underlying cause for poor weight gain in the baby and/or a low milk supply, other factors need to be ruled out as discussed in Chapter 3. More information on pumps can be found here www.sarahoakleylactation.co.uk/choosing-a-breast-pump.

Not everyone will be able to express enough milk to meet their baby's needs, at least not initially. Expressing, like breastfeeding, is a learned skill and takes practice and our bodies simply do not respond to a pump in the same way as they do to a baby. When you hold your baby close, feel their warm breath on your skin, look into their eyes and smell their skin this stimulates the release of oxytocin and the milk begins to flow. A plastic pump with its grinding motor does not have the same effect. Warming up the breasts with hot flannels or a warm shower and massaging the breasts before expressing can be helpful, as well as keeping baby close and using relaxation techniques including breathing, meditation, imagery, and visualisation. These can all 'trick' your body into releasing the magical oxytocin and with repetition of these triggers you can condition your body to respond to the pump.

Galactagogues are medications and herbal supplements that can help enhance the effects of breastfeeding and expressing and increase milk supply. Which ones are right and safe for you will depend on why your supply is low, your medical history and any other medications you are taking. An IBCLC and a medical herbalist are usually best placed to discuss your options, in conjunction with your GP. The book *Making More Milk* by Lisa Marasco and Diana West has detailed information on galactagogues and foods that may help increase supply.

If you cannot express enough milk to meet your baby's needs, you will need to use donor milk or formula. Donor milk is only available via NHS milk banks to premature and sick babies on the NICU. However, the Hearts Milk Bank, based near Welwyn Garden City in Hertfordshire, will supply donor milk to families who do not meet the NHS criteria, so depending on your circumstances this can be worth exploring. Their website is heartsmilkbank.org.

Informal milk sharing is another route to accessing donor milk. However, in this situation the donor isn't screened for health issues and the milk is not tested for infection, or pasteurised, as it is in the NHS and the Hearts Milk Bank. So caution needs to be exercised and it is advisable to pasteurise the milk yourself at home prior to use. Human Milk for Human Babies has a Facebook page which puts donors and recipients in touch and provides support with informal milk sharing.

Whether using donor milk or formula the amounts given at each feed, whether as a full feed or a top-up alongside a breastfeed, need to be appropriate. Healthcare professionals regularly overestimate the volumes babies require, especially newborns, and the volumes quoted on the side of formula packaging are too large as they are based on fewer feeds than a breastfed baby would normally take. Over-feeding is an issue because it can make babies uncomfortable and contribute to reflux. It can also mean that babies wake less often to feed, which means less breast stimulation and a further reduced milk supply. In the first 24 hours of life a baby will take around a teaspoon (5ml) of colostrum at each feed, yet mums are often told to give babies at this stage 30ml of formula per feed. Feed volume gradually increases to around 60ml per feed at day seven and 90ml by day 14. If a baby is going to the breast and taking some milk, but not enough, then starting top-ups at half the full feed volume and monitoring weight so these can be adjusted seems sensible in the first couple of weeks and is my usual approach. However, for older babies with slow gain starting with a total top-up volume of 120ml in 24 hours and then titrating this against weight gain can be a good way to avoid over-feeding and protect the milk supply while addressing the need for additional calories.

The method by which any supplement is given can have an impact on breastfeeding. It is very easy to overfeed with a bottle as babies tend to take these more quickly than a breastfeed and this can interfere with feelings of fullness and leave a baby unsettled due to tummy discomfort from drinking too quickly. This unsettledness can lead parents to think their baby is still hungry and offer more. Furthermore, a baby will end a breastfeed with non-nutritive sucking (comfort sucking) which helps them to settle to sleep. A bottle-fed baby cannot replicate this on an empty bottle so will require settling in other ways. For breastfed babies having top-ups from a bottle offering the breast after the top-up can help with settling. But the most important consideration with offering bottles to any baby, even if they are fully bottle-fed, is pacing the feed. This will also help prevent the baby becoming lazy when returned to the breast.

Paced feeding involves sitting your baby upright for feeds and teasing the lips with the bottle teat until the baby opens their mouth wide and then placing the bottle teat in the mouth. The bottle is held horizontally and tilted slightly so milk fills the teat. This slows the flow and means the baby must work to draw the milk as they would at the breast. Periodically the parent pauses the flow by tilting the bottle teat upwards into the roof of the mouth or withdrawing the teat onto the lip to break the seal. This pausing mimics normal breastfeeding behaviour and ensures that a feed is taken over a 10–20-minute period and not guzzled down in five minutes flat.

But are bottles the only or best option for a baby who is going to be breastfed? The answer to both questions is 'no'. For newborns syringe-feeding while the baby sucks on the parent's index finger (finger pad facing up towards the roof of the mouth) or cup-feeding will avoid nipple confusion and any negative impact on the latch. For babies that are starting to need volumes larger than about 30ml finger-feeding using an infant nasogastric feeding tube dangled into a bottle of breastmilk or formula and placed at the tip of the finger the baby is to suck on, or a lactation aid, is preferable. A lactation aid (or supplementary nursing system) involves placing a tube at the nipple so that when the baby is latched on and feeding, they takes their supplement via the tube while continuing to feed at the breast. A lactation aid can be made from a normal feeding bottle and infant nasogastric feeding tube or you can buy a Medela Supplementary Nursing System. Jack Newman, a Canadian paediatrician, has information on his website about lactation aids: ibconline.ca/information-sheets/lactation-aid.

Having seen a non-latching tongue-tied baby completely lose the ability to suck after ten days of cup feeding without any opportunity to suck, I am cautious about the use of exclusive cup-feeding beyond the first couple of days.

Finger-feeding can be useful in training babies to suck more effectively. It can help to improve tongue tone and placement and the sucking action used by the baby is like the sucking action the baby will use at the breast. Finger-feeding can be a useful way to transition a non-latching baby to the breast. It also means a partner can be involved and share the load when a mother finds herself having to breastfeed, top-up and express.

The lactation aid has the advantage of ensuring maximum stimulation at the breast and can reduce the need for expressing. It also helps to teach the baby to feed more effectively at the breast and avoids any of the drawbacks of the other methods. Babies also tend to regulate their intake with this method.

As with expressing it is vital to access support from an IBCLC or other professional to work out the best method for feeding your baby while you are establishing breastfeeding and managing any concerns about weight gain and low supply.

Breast compression

A final feeding strategy which can help a baby whose efficiency at the breast is compromised by a tongue-tie or in the early days after division is breast compression. It is also helpful when shields are being used. Your baby latches on to the breast and feeds through the initial 'let down'. When the flow starts to subside and your baby shows signs of working harder with more frequent pausing, less swallowing and is in danger of falling asleep due to fatigue, you take a large handful of breast with your thumb opposite your fingers and compress the breast firmly and continuously. Your hand should be placed halfway between the nipple and the ribcage and the continuous compression (or squeezing) should be applied when your baby is sucking and released when they pause. The compression creates more flow and simulates another 'let down', making it easier for your baby to remove milk from the breast. If this is working the baby will start to suck and swallow more vigorously again, and become more alert if they had started to drift off to sleep. When this compression is no longer effective it is time to swap breasts.

Tummy time

As explained in Chapter 3 tongue-ties can cause jaw tension and the process of birth can leave babies with tensions and strains in their jaw, neck and back, which may impact feeding. Input from a body worker (osteopath, chiropractor or cranial sacral therapist) may be helpful before and after tongue-tie division, and for babies who are not going to have a division. This is something to discuss with your tongue-tie practitioner. But a simple thing parents can do, which can also help rebalance the muscles in the neck area, is tummy time. All babies benefit from tummy time as it helps to prevent flattening of the back of the head and strengthens the spine ready for sitting. It is not safe for babies to sleep on their tummies, as this has been shown to increase the risk of SIDS. However, it is safe to do when baby is awake and supervised. Some babies may struggle with being on their tummies at first, so start with short sessions of a minute or two. Supporting your baby's shoulders on a rolled-up towel, or draping them over a firm nursing or V-shaped pillow so their head is off the floor initially, can help to get them used to being on their front. Aim for a few short sessions a day.

What about bottle-fed babies?

We have already looked at paced feeding and how this can reduce overfeeding, wind, and reflux symptoms. Bottle-fed babies also often struggle to form a seal on a bottle teat and create a vacuum to draw milk. There are many different types of botte teats on the market. Some are long, some are short and stubby, some are wedge-shaped or flat, some are rounded. Some are broad and fit to a wide-neck bottle, while some are narrower and fit to the more traditional bottle shape. They are often made of silicone nowadays. But latex teats are still available, and some teats come in both silicone and latex options. It is often necessary to experiment to find out what best suits your baby.

The high palate associated with a tongue-tie can trigger an over-active gag reflex, so a shorter teat may suit these babies better. Wedge-shaped or flatter teats may also help to fill this palate space and create a better seal for some babies. Some babies seem to get a better seal on a latex teat. Smaller babies will often do better on the narrower teats. Experimenting with flow rates is also sensible. A baby who is struggling to drain a bottle may do better on a faster flow teat. But equally a baby who is gulping and choking on the bottle may need a slower flow teat. There is no single bottle teat design which will suit all babies and it can get expensive trying different options, so buy just one at a time and not a pack of six. Change to a different shape teat, or from silicone to latex, rather than trying different teats that are similar.

Support for you

Having a baby who is struggling to feed can be exhausting,

demoralising and a source of great anxiety. It can take time to work out what is causing the difficulties and to get the right help with resolving them. The idea of having a tongue-tie division which will 'fix' everything is perpetuated on social media and by some less well-informed professionals and it is an attractive idea for parents. But tongue-tie division is rarely an instant fix and some of the difficulty you may be facing may not be tongue-tie related at all. I see many mothers and babies who struggle in the early weeks where the baby does not have a tongue-tie. They need help over a period of several weeks to establish and feel confident with breastfeeding. This is to be expected.

Breastfeeding is a learned skill for parents and the transition to parenthood causes huge practical, emotional and psychological upheaval. Life will never 'get back to normal'. The birth of a baby means a fundamental irreversible change has happened and that takes some adjusting to.

Families need support. However, certainly in the UK, we see fewer families with local extended family support available and parents can find themselves very isolated. Midwifery and health visiting services are under resourced, with the number of routine visits reduced over the last two decades, so help from these sources may be difficult to access. The availability of specialist infant feeding support from the NHS is highly variable depending on where you live.

Ideally the person who divides your baby's tongue-tie should be an IBCLC or work with an IBCLC, or be able to put you in touch with ongoing specialist breastfeeding support, so you can access skilled follow-up help in the weeks after division. But this is not always the case.

So, it is important to try to seek out support and, in most areas, there will be free breastfeeding support groups you can access. At the time of writing this book we are in the middle of the Coronavirus pandemic and one good thing to perhaps come out of this, from a breastfeeding support perspective, is the increase in availability of online support. There has never been any consistency in the availability of local breastfeeding support, with some groups being commissioned and paid for by the NHS or local authorities and others run by charities and volunteers. Austerity has seen many funded groups cut. Some areas are much better served than others as a result. With online support geography is not a barrier and it can also make it easier to access help on those days when everything is just too overwhelming to get out of your pyjamas. Many lactation consultants and breastfeeding counsellors are offering one-to-one sessions online too. You can find out what is on offer in your area via your midwife or health visitor, your local children's centre, online mum and baby groups, and social media. Charities such as the NCT, Association of Breastfeeding Mothers, Breastfeeding Network and La Leche League have trained volunteer peer supporters and breastfeeding counsellors who offer helplines, email and online chat support, and can direct you to local support groups run by their volunteers or others.

Breastfeeding is a relationship which develops and changes between parent and baby over time. Feeding patterns and behaviours change, sleep patterns change, and rate of growth changes as babies get older. There are also huge normal variations in when individual babies meet developmental milestones. These changes can be a source of anxiety for parents and many of the queries I receive relate to completely normal behaviours. It is normal for babies to spit up small amounts of milk. It is normal for babies to have unsettled periods. It is normal for them to want to be held and comforted and not want to sleep alone. It is normal for them to feed frequently and wake frequently. Talking to other mothers helps to normalise all this.

Having a network of people who are 'in your corner' is extremely helpful. As well as healthcare professionals and breastfeeding supporters this can include friends and family who are supportive of your goals and may include 'online' or 'virtual' friends. Many parents find accessing parenting and breastfeeding groups on platforms such as Facebook creates new friendships and provides a safe space to discuss worries and ask for information. Some parents find employing a postnatal doula extremely valuable, especially when family support is limited or not available. Doula UK provides information on what a doula can offer and has a directory of doulas to help you find someone suitable. They also have an access fund for those families in financial hardship. Their website is doula.org.uk.

These national charities provide free breastfeeding support via helplines, email, social media and face-to-face in group and one-to-one settings:

- Association of Breastfeeding Mothers www.abm.me.uk
- Breastfeeding Network www.breastfeedingnetwork.org.uk
- La Leche League GB www.laleche.org.uk

Specialist support

In some cases, the feeding difficulties your baby is experiencing are not going to be entirely related to a tongue-tie. Even after a division some babies will continue to struggle. As already discussed, many babies benefit from body work, especially those that have had traumatic births. But some babies need more. They may have issues with muscle tone, co-ordination and sensory processing, which may relate to developmental or neurological issues. They may have physical health problems such as a heart defect or laryngomalacia (floppy larynx) that is impacting their feeding. While some conditions and health problems will be identified at birth or even before birth, many developmental and neurological conditions may not be evident at birth and will emerge and be diagnosed later. Early feeding issues that are difficult to resolve may be the first sign that there is a problem.

Many experienced IBCLCs will be able to offer support with feeding babies who have issues with low or high muscle tone, or sensory integration difficulties. Strategies may include suck training, exercises to improve tongue mobility and positioning and latching techniques. But in many cases input from other disciplines including speech and language therapy, paediatrics, ENT, physiotherapy, and occupational therapy will be required.

However, in most cases infant feeding issues can be resolved with a short period of skilled help.

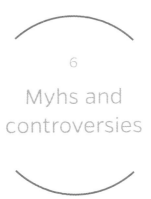

6

Myhs and
controversies

Hop on to any Facebook group on infant tongue-tie and you will see posts about lip tie. Parents flip up their baby's top lip and what do they see? A membrane attaching the top lip to the upper gum. Surely this is the key to the feeding issues they have been experiencing. But is it? What exactly is a lip tie?

The presence of a frenulum (a tethering) stretching from the upper gum to behind the upper lip in the midline is normal anatomy according to the dental literature (Mohan et al, 2014). A study conducted at the Louisiana State University Health Science Center School of Dentistry (Townsend et al, 2013) describes this tethering as follows:

The median maxillary labial frenum (MMLF) is a fold of mucous membrane found on the underside of the center of the upper lip that connects to the midline of the attached gingiva between the central incisors. It adapts to any of the normal movements of the lip. As the primary teeth erupt, the height in the alveolar structures increases normally and the attachment of the frenum moves superiorly with the maxillary alveolar crest.

So crucially the upper labial frenulum adapts to the normal movements of the lip and its point of attachment will gradually move up the gum once the first teeth come in.

So where does the idea of a restricted upper labial frenulum or 'lip tie' come from? The answer is dental practitioners in the USA. Larry Kotlow (2015) has created a classification system for what he calls 'upper lip tie' based on the appearance of the upper labial frenulum. Interest in the upper labial frenulum seems to have started with concerns regarding the impact a frenulum that is attached low on the upper gum may have from a dental perspective. In the USA many tongue-tie divisions in infants are carried out by dentists. There seems to have been a move towards dividing the upper labial frenulum, at the same time as the tongue-tie, to avoid dental decay and diastema (a gap between the front teeth) as the child grows up.

A misunderstanding of the role of the upper lip in breastfeeding then appears to have led to the idea that the upper labial frenulum may create feeding difficulties. As Larry Kotlow (2015) writes:

When the upper lip's inner mucosa is attached to the alveolar ridge of the maxillary arch and the lip is unable to fully flange upward, it also can also become a factor in creating a shallow latch.

However, a study involving 11 infants using real-time MRI to image the breastfeeding swallow found that eight of the infants had their upper lip in a neutral position during latch, two had it in an everted position and in the remaining infant lip position could not be accurately determined (Mills et al, 2020). None were fully flanged.

This is because the upper lip does not need to fully flange to achieve a deep latch. In fact an overly flanged upper lip is a sign of a problem. Catherine Watson Genna, a well-known and respected American IBCLC, writes in her book *Supporting Sucking Skills in the Breastfeeding Infant* (3rd Edition, 2017):

> *The upper lip should be neutral to slightly everted on the breast and should be relatively immobile during feeding.*

> *An overly flanged upper lip is a sign of a shallow attachment or overuse of the lip to compensate for tongue immobility.*

The second point explains why both professionals and parents may perceive an improvement in latch following lip tie division. The added ability to fully flange the top lip, following a lip tie division, will allow a baby to compensate for continued poor positioning or tongue function issues. But of course, this is treating a symptom and not the underlying cause and does not justify unnecessary surgery. Improving positioning, tongue-tie division, tongue exercises and suck training to promote effective tongue mobility would be more appropriate.

One major issue with lip tie division and claims that it improves feeding is that it is frequently carried out at the same time as tongue-tie division. So how do we know the feeding wouldn't have improved simply by dividing the tongue-tie and leaving the lip alone? At the annual conference of The Australasian Society for Tongue and Lip Ties in 2019, Holly Puckering (a speech and language pathologist) spoke about an audit carried out in her clinic on infants with feeding difficulties. They stopped dividing lip ties routinely alongside tongue-tie division and focused on normalising tongue function first, achieving a reduction in lip tie division from 22% to 1.3% over a three-year period with no adverse impact on long-term outcomes. This suggests that many of the lip tie divisions they had been doing were unnecessary.

The bottom line is that there is no research to support lip tie division in babies to improve feeding. A systematic review of the medical literature published in 2019 (Nakhesh et al) concluded that 'the evidence for routine upper lip tie release in infants with breastfeeding difficulties is poor'. But might it still be a good idea to prevent dental issues as the child gets older?

Alison Hazelbaker, IBCLC (author of the Hazelbaker Assessment Tool for Lingual Frenulum Function discussed earlier in this book) writes in her blog 'Modern Myths about Tongue-tie: The Unnecessary Controversy Continues':

> *The assertion that dental caries is caused by an upper lip tie begs to be proven. Breastmilk does not pool in the mouth. The position of the nipple in the mouth and the manner in which that milk is moved into the pharynx for the swallow will not allow it. Both the peristaltic action of the tongue and the pressure differential created by tongue movements quickly push/pull the milk to its ultimate destination.*

I have not been able to find anything in the literature to support an association between upper lip ties and dental decay, or indeed speech.

Furthermore, concerns have been raised about complications arising from division of 'lip ties' in babies. Unlike tongue-tie division, which is a long-established procedure in babies, lip tie divisions have only been carried out within the last 15 years or so. There are anecdotal reports of babies not latching following lip tie division due to pain and discomfort. The upper labial frenulum is much more sensitive and vascular than the lingual frenulum. Angus Cameron, an Associate Professor of Dentistry in Australia, explained to me in a telephone conversation in 2015 that he had come across cases where the adult teeth inside the gum had been damaged during the procedure and where scar tissue formation had created a permanent diastema. He has this information on his website (sydneytonguetie.com.au):

> There is currently NO evidence that a thick or short labial frenum has any negative influence on breast-feeding. The mere presence of a labial frenum does NOT indicate a need for surgery.
>
> Releasing an upper labial frenum is a traumatic procedure that may also lead to more dental problems later including the persistence of an anterior diastema (gap between the front teeth) that is difficult to close orthodontically.

In the UK, in the rare cases where an upper labial frenulum remains attached low on the gum and will cause a diastema when the adult teeth emerge, division may be offered at around 10–12 years.

Discussions on social media can make this a very confusing issue for parents. Alongside lip tie you may also find mention of buccal tie. Buccal ties are the membranes (frenula) that stretch between our cheeks and upper gums. Like the labial and lingual frenula, they are normal anatomy. From what we know about how a baby latches and feeds, there is nothing to suggest these should be divided to improve feeding. There is nothing in the research that I have been able to find that even mentions buccal tie in relation to feeding difficulties in babies. According to Linda D'Onofiro (2019), pronounced buccal ties may act as a pocket for food, which of course may lead to dental decay. My advice would be to discuss any concerns you have with your dentist.

I find it worrying that when tongue-tie division has not yielded the improvements parents and practitioners would like, we look for something else to cut.

Tongue-tie and speech

One of the most common concerns parents have with regards to tongue-tie is whether it will cause difficulties with speech later if left untreated. Most of the available research on tongue-tie focuses on breastfeeding. Little can be found on tongue-tie in relation to speech. So how might a tongue-tie impact speech? Mags Kirk, an independent speech and language therapist, explains:

We know that the NICE guidelines specify that a tongue-tie should only be divided if it is affecting an infant's feeding. But what if it doesn't get cut at a young age and then poses a problem with speech development later on? In my experience children with undivided tongue-ties may go on to have speech articulation problems in the future. It's not a guarantee though, and of course, your child might end up with speech problems regardless of whether they have a tongue-tie or not.

So, what are the main issues I see? Well, I have found that speech and feeding development are intrinsically linked. Think about the way that the tongue develops for feeding from birth. A healthy full-term baby is born with the ability to suckle, and so they learn to suck from the breast or a bottle. The suck gradually gets stronger, and so the baby becomes more efficient at feeding.

At the age of six months, weaning foods are commonly introduced, and now the tongue learns lateral, side-to-side movements, because it needs to move the food around the mouth so that it can be chewed. This lateral movement is absolutely essential as it needs to develop before tongue tip elevation can occur. Tongue tip elevation is a crucial part of how most consonant speech sounds are made.

The stability of the tongue in the mouth is crucial for clear development. Try this:

Close your eyes, then count out loud from number one through to twenty while focusing on what your tongue is doing in your mouth. What did you notice? Think about how many times the sides of your tongue touch your top molar teeth. It happens on practically every word and is particularly apparent when you get into the teen words for the 'ee' sound. The place where your tongue goes for the 'ee' sound is how your tongue gets stability. Without tongue stability it is impossible for the tongue tip to move to where it needs to go to articulate clearly.

Children with untreated tongue-tie are frequently unable to achieve this tongue stability. They start to move their tongue in all sorts of ways to get stability. Some children will develop an open mouth posture with their tongue slightly out of their mouth. Some will be able to keep their mouth closed, but the tongue will remain in a downwards posture in their mouth, rather than where the tongue should live, resting on the palate, on the roof of the mouth.

So why is tongue resting posture important? Well, if an incorrect tongue resting posture is formed, this has an impact on how the tongue can move for specific speech sounds. Think of all the sounds in English that need the tongue tip to elevate… t, d, s, z, sh, ch, j, l, n, and r. If the tongue is in a low resting posture because of a tongue-tie, it makes it hard for the tongue to be able to elevate to the spot just behind the top teeth to make these sounds. The sounds might come out sounding slushy, or distorted. The child might end up having a lisp – either a frontal *lisp where the 's' and 'z' sounds become like a 'th', or a lateral lisp, where the air comes out of the sides of the mouth rather than the front, resulting in a sound a little like the Welsh 'll'.*

Tongue-tie can also play havoc with the 'r' sound. For the correct production of the 'r', the tongue needs the back of tongue stability we discussed above when thinking about the 'ee' sound, but also it needs tension within the tongue muscles. Try this: make a long 'rrrrr' sound, keeping your tongue tight and the tongue tip up to the roof of the mouth. Now relax the sides of your tongue but keep your tongue tip up to the palate. You might notice that the sound becomes more like a 'w' sound. Children with tongue-tie might have difficulty with the tongue tip elevation, but they can also struggle with getting the side tongue muscles nice and tight to get the correct 'r' sound.

The 'l' sound can also be problematic. If a child has a tongue-tie, they might be able to get the 'ee' back of tongue stability, but they might not be able to elevate their tongue tip. The result – often the child will say a 'w' or a 'y' sound instead.

I find it interesting that even adults can continue to experience articulation problems. Some adults have even cashed in on their speech problem – think of Jonathan Ross's 'r' sound, or Drew Barrymore's lisp.

Most childhood articulation difficulties clear up eventually as the child matures, but some adults continue to have problems with their 's' 'r' and 'l' sounds. I would be interested to look in these adults' mouths to spot whether they have an untreated tongue-tie. In most cases where I have been able to have a look, I have found the answer to be a definite yes.

A Japanese paper from 2015 (Ito et al) looked at the effectiveness of division in five children aged 3–8 years with articulation difficulties. The results were mixed, with some early improvement seen in omission and substitutions of sounds in the first 3–4 months post-division, but ongoing issues with distortion noted at 1–2 years. A study in the USA by Richard Baxter and colleagues (2020) reported on a sample of 37 children aged 13 months to 12 years, in which 89% showed improvements in speech after one month, but there was no long term follow-up. However, both studies are severely limited by their small sample size, the lack of a control group, and the lack of comparison with other interventions such as speech therapy which could be as effective, or more effective, than surgery.

Interestingly, another small study looking at 59 children aged two years one month to four years 11 months found no significant differences between those children that had had division as babies, had a tongue-tie but had not had division, and those that had never had a tongue-tie (Salt et al, 2020). They measured frenulum structure and function, tongue mobility and speech production and intelligibility. The authors concluded:

> *This study provides preliminary evidence of no difference between tongue mobility and speech outcomes in young children with or without intervention for tongue-tie during infancy. This study assists with clinical decision making and makes recommendations for families not to proceed with surgical intervention for tongue-tie during infancy, for the sole outcome of improving speech production later in life.*

This conclusion supports the stance adopted in the UK when it comes to tongue-tie division, which is to only divide the frenulum if it seems to be causing a significant feeding difficulty. This can be a source of anxiety for parents worried about speech. But as this study shows, having a division may not result in significant differences in tongue function and speech in the long term. As we saw in Chapter 4 the Z plasty division procedure combined with myotomy (release of the genioglossus muscle) when the child is older may provide better results in terms of resolving speech issues (Choi et al, 2011).

There is also the possibility that the tongue-tie will reoccur over time. Research on wound healing suggests that the wound may remodel over a period of two years, so recurrence many months or even a year or two down the line is possible. Plus, we also need to keep in mind that impaired tongue tip elevation is a significant factor in speech difficulties, as Mags explained earlier. But babies with significant restriction in tongue elevation are likely to have significant feeding issues, particularly in terms of weight gain and efficiency, so are highly likely to fall into the criteria for division for feeding anyway. Finally, of course, division is not without potential complications and can disrupt breastfeeding, even if only briefly, and this is not something we would want to risk based on preventing an issue that may never arise.

Tongue-tie and dental issues

A lack of tongue mobility, particularly lateral (side-to-side) movement may make it difficult to clear food debris away from teeth and spread saliva, predisposing to dental decay.

Tongue posture and function influences the growth and development of bony structures of the oral cavity including the palate and jaw. 'The shortness of the lingual frenum can affect the physiological posture of the tongue and its neuromuscular behaviour' (Dezio et al, 2015). The low tongue posture and tongue thrust associated with a tongue-tie can cause malocclusion, such as an open bite and spreading of the lower front teeth (Vaz & Bai, 2015, Jang et al, 2011, and Dezio et al, 2015).

So, should tongue-tie division be offered to babies and young children to prevent dental problems later? Paediatric surgeon Paul Johnson (2006) writes:

Problems with dentition have been reported with tongue-tie including lower incisor deformity, gingival recession, and malocclusions. However, the evidence is not strong enough to recommend prophylactic division of tongue-tie in order to prevent malocclusion. Often these conditions are associated with additional abnormalities such as deviation of the epiglottis or larynx. It is widely accepted that the tongue can influence face development and cases of impaired maxillary and mandibular development being resolved by tongue-tie division have been reported.

Clearly, as with feeding and speech, the impact of tongue-tie on dentition needs further research. But dental concerns may be a reason for division of tongue-tie to be considered in older children and adults. For babies, the over-riding concern when it comes to tongue-tie is the impact it can have on feeding.

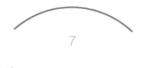

7

When treatment
doesn't improve
things

On the face of it, the idea that a simple snip of the lingual frenulum can end the misery of shredded nipples, the anxiety of a baby who is not gaining weight, the exhaustion associated with a baby who needs to feed continuously or is permanently unhappy due to the discomfort of reflux is an attractive one. Most parents would, understandably, grasp this opportunity with both hands.

But of course, it is not as simple as that. As we have seen, there are potential complications to consider and outcomes are not guaranteed. Other factors can be impacting on feeding and these need to be addressed to optimise the chances of a successful outcome after division.

In offering to divide a tongue-tie in a baby with a feeding difficulty, practitioners are offering an opportunity to improve feeding. But the stakes can feel high. As a parent you are making a decision to put your baby through what is widely regarded as a minor, safe surgical procedure. But there is a risk your baby will experience some pain and potentially struggle with feeding in the early days after division, perhaps more so than before. Complications are rare but the risks of bleeding, infection and damage to other oral structures sound scary, and then there is the risk of recurrence and the thought of maybe having to go through it all again. Consenting to division is an act of faith and you are placing your trust completely in the practitioner. For the practitioner, the sense of responsibility can weigh heavy.

We all want a swift, successful outcome. However much I prepare parents, telling them not to expect a quick fix, and explaining that there are other factors we need to work on and that this will all take a bit of time and commitment, I am still secretly hoping for an early and straightforward resolution to the feeding problems, otherwise what sort of a practitioner am I?

As a parent you are making a difficult decision, often at a stressful time in the early days of parenting with the added pressure of a baby who is not feeding well. You do not know what day of the week it is or even what time it is, yet you have to weigh up the pros and cons of putting your baby through a surgical procedure. Of course, you want and expect the best outcome.

But what happens when division does *not* result in improvement in feeding, not just in the short term, but in the long term? How does that feel?

From a practitioner perspective it can be very frustrating, disappointing, and undermining. Often parents arrive at our door after a long and torturous journey involving weeks or even months of challenges, poor information and sometimes well-meaning but ineffective support. They are broken and they simply do not have the physical, emotional, and mental resources left to persevere and wait for improvements after division. It can also be emotionally and mentally challenging to provide ongoing support to families where improvement in feeding is going to take several weeks, especially when it is not always obvious why feeding remains a challenge. There is an overwhelming feeling that having done the division you are exclusively responsible for ensuring a positive outcome. You have to have all the answers. When things are not going smoothly, or progress is slow or erratic, you question whether the division was justified. Did you do a good division? Have you missed something? Do you have the skills needed to help these parents?

As a parent you may have similar questions. Was it right to do the division? Was the division done properly? Was the division done too late? Is it hopeless? Can I continue? Is it worth it? Have I put my baby through this for nothing? Will my baby have longer term problems with feeding or speech? What if this happens with my next baby?

I spoke to two mothers about their experiences of tongue-tie division without the desired outcome. Their stories are shared below:

Lucy's story

Lucy, a second-time mum who was working as a breastfeeding peer supporter at the time, told me about her son Oliver who had a division at day four and then wouldn't latch to the breast for 18 weeks afterwards. Lucy was desperate to breastfeed Oliver after a difficult feeding journey with her first baby. So when Oliver struggled to latch, and a posterior tongue-tie was identified, she insisted on having it divided as soon as possible. When he then refused to latch and seemed to develop an aversion to the breast Lucy felt rejected by her baby and a failure as a mum. Now, some years later, and having qualified as an IBCLC, Lucy believes she should have waited and not gone ahead with division so early on. However, at the time she says she could not acknowledge that her decision to divide may have made things worse. After unsuccessful attempts to get Oliver to latch and feed with shields and the use of a lactation aid Lucy resigned herself to pumping and bottle-feeding. She focused on skin-to-skin and cuddles at the breast to start to build a positive relationship with the breast for Oliver. After a further four weeks, with the pressure to breastfeed reduced, Oliver just suddenly latched one day and fed. Lucy still had the challenge of an oversupply to overcome, induced by the constant pumping, and Oliver would only latch in the underarm hold standing up at first, but ultimately she achieved her goal of exclusively breastfeeding him.

Nicola's story

Nicola's first baby, Chloe, was born early at 35 weeks weighing just 5lb. She never latched. As a first-time mum Nicola expected there to be help and support with establishing breastfeeding but there wasn't. She would spend 30 minutes trying to latch Chloe on and then she would express and bottle-feed her. She went through this lengthy, exhausting, and disheartening process eight times a day, every day. At six weeks Nicola realised Chloe might be tongue-tied and sought help privately. Chloe's tongue-tie was divided but she still didn't latch, and Nicola continued the three-hourly cycle of expressing and bottle-feeding. She missed out on holding Chloe as her partner took over most of the feeding so Nicola could pump. She didn't sleep for months and could no longer think clearly. She would cry when washing out the bottles *and felt let down by everyone she had had contact with. There was simply not enough support. In describing her experience Nicola told me, 'there is nothing wrong with formula, but you lose something'. Nicola's experience left her so traumatised that she needed therapy and even now, nine years later, she still feels deeply about it and cried during our conversation. Nicola went on to have another baby and was petrified this baby wouldn't feed and had to make sure she had access to breastfeeding support. Her baby had a tongue-tie identified and treated early on and successfully breastfed and this sounds like it helped to heal some of the old wounds.*

Professor Amy Brown has researched the issue of breastfeeding trauma and explores this in her book *Why Breastfeeding Grief and Trauma Matter*, which I would recommend parents and those supporting them read. I have certainly seen many parents who have been left traumatised by the feeding difficulties they experienced in relation to tongue-tie. These feelings of trauma I would argue stem from not feeling listened to when feeding is problematic, the long and arduous journey to diagnosis and treatment, and then the disappointment when treatment outcomes do not meet expectations. The legacy of this trauma is always, in my experience, seen when the next baby comes along. Mothers are haunted by their previous experience. I have mothers contacting me in the first trimester of their next pregnancy to explore my availability to see them as soon as the baby is born. I have had mothers in this situation come to my clinic on their way home from hospital, when their baby is literally only a few hours old, to have them checked for tongue-tie. I have treated two babies at 17 hours old. Both were second babies, and both were not latching after birth. Their mothers had had difficulties breastfeeding their older siblings and tongue-tie diagnosis had been delayed. They were not taking any chances the second time round. However, with early support, treatment, and diagnosis these mothers often remain highly anxious about feeding, even in cases where the second baby isn't tongue-tied.

In some cases, this anxiety becomes overwhelming and threatens the new breastfeeding relationship. I have supported some mothers who have not been able to separate out the two experiences. When asked about the birth and feeding issues they talk about their previous experience, sometimes at greater length than the current experience. They sometimes talk about both babies simultaneously, mixing up the names, so it can be quite hard to follow whether what is being described is a current issue or a past issue. They are literally haunted by their past experience and this can easily sabotage the current one. It can be very difficult to set aside the previous experience and see the new baby as a different child, a different experience and a new relationship.

Skilled and timely feeding support remains vital, but as Lucy told me, having access to great support, as she did, carries no guarantees. I think mothers needs more than that. You need honesty and information. You need choices and to feel safe. You need to feel listened to and above all you need to be heard. This is why Nicola, and others, have shared their experiences in this book. I hope that it is helpful.

If you are struggling as the result of your feeding experience then please do seek help. Breastfeeding counsellors, IBCLCs and doulas all offer support and debriefing and can help you prepare for the next baby. Your health visitor and GP can also provide help managing grief and anxiety.

Appendix

Summary of some of the research that has looked at the efficacy of tongue-tie division in infants.

Berry, J., Griffiths, M., Westcott, C. A double-blind, randomised controlled trial of tongue-tie division and its immediate effect on breastfeeding. *Breastfeeding Medicine*, 2012, 7: 189-193.
- Double-blind sham-controlled RCT, with adequate concealment, similar groups and subjects analysed into groups they were allocated to. N=60 (57 completed).
- Outcome 1. 78% (21) of mothers in intervention group reported improved feeding compared to 47% (14) of the placebo group, (P<0.02). This was evidence that the placebo effect alone did not account for the difference in reported outcomes.

Hogan, M., Westcott, C., Griffiths, M. A randomised, controlled trial of division of tongue-tie in infants with feeding problems. *Journal of Paediatrics and Child Health*; 2005.
- 57 babies with tongue-tie; 40 were breastfed and 17 were bottle-fed: 28 had tongue-tie divided (20 breastfed and 8 bottle-fed) 29 controls did not have tongue-tie divided (20 breastfed, 9 bottle-fed).
- Mean age = 20 days (range 3 to 70)
- Improvement within 48 hours: Division group = 96% (27/28) Control group = 3% (1/29) p <0.001
- Improvement within 48 hours for breastfed babies: Division group = 95% (19/20) Control group = 5% (1/20) p <0.001
- The remaining 28 mothers in the control group all subsequently requested tongue-tie division. After the procedure, 96% (27/28) of babies improved (all within 48 hours, except for one baby who improved after 7 days).
- Overall improved feeding = 95% (54/57)

Buryk, M., Bloom, D., Shope, T. Efficacy of neonatal release of ankyloglossia: a randomized trial. Pediatrics, 2011; 128: 280-286.
- Single-blinded sham-controlled RCT, with adequate concealment, similar groups and subjects analysed into groups they were allocated to. N=58
- Both the sham and intervention groups reported significant improvement in nipple pain immediately after the procedure, but there was still a significant improvement between the intervention and sham treatment groups (<0.001).

Alan Emond et al. Randomised controlled trial of early frenotomy in breastfed infants with mild–moderate tongue-tie. *BMJ*, Volume 99, Issue 3, 2013.

- A randomised, parallel group, pragmatic trial, babies aged 0–2 weeks, mild or moderate degree of tongue-tie.
- 107 infants were randomised, 55 to the intervention group and 52 to the comparison group.
- Frenotomy did improve the tongue-tie and increased maternal breastfeeding self-efficacy. At 5 days, there was a 15.5% increase in bottle-feeding in the comparison group compared with a 7.5% increase in the intervention group.
- Early frenotomy did not result in an objective improvement in breastfeeding but was associated with improved self-efficacy. The majority in the comparison arm opted for the intervention after 5 days.

O'Callahan, C., Macary, S., Clemente, S. (2013) The effects of office-based frenotomy for anterior and posterior ankyloglossia on breastfeeding. *International Journal of Pediatric Otorhinolaryngology* 77 (2013) 827–832.

- Women whose infants underwent a frenotomy from December 2006 through March 2011 were asked to complete an 18-item, web-based questionnaire about maternal-infant breastfeeding characteristics before and after the intervention. The web-linked questionnaire was offered between December 2010 and May 2011.
- There were 311 infants evaluated for ankyloglossia and 299 (95%) underwent a frenotomy. Most infants were classified as having Type III (36%) or IV (49%) ankyloglossia compared to only 16% with anterior (Type I and Type II combined).
- Among survey respondents (n = 157), infant latching significantly improved (P <.001) from pre- to post-intervention for infants with posterior ankyloglossia. Both the presence and severity of nipple pain decreased from pre- to post-intervention among all classifications (P <.001). Additionally, 92% of respondents breastfed exclusively post-intervention. The mean breastfeeding duration of 14 months did not differ significantly by classification.

Ghaheri, B., Cole, M., Fausel, S., Chuop, M., Mace, J. Breastfeeding improvement following tongue-tie and lip-tie release: A prospective cohort study. *Laryngoscope*, September 2016. http://onlinelibrary.wiley.com/doi/10.1002/lary.26306/full

- 700 babies age 0–12 weeks, LC support and assessment pre- and post-division, follow-up one week, one month and again at six months to check for reattachment.

- Follow-up looked at self-efficacy, pain scores, reflux, milk transfer (test weighs).
- 237 babies in results: 25% tongue-tie, 75% tongue-tie and lip tie, 0.4% lip tie.
- 3% needed re-division.
- 22% anterior, 78% posterior.
- All showed improvement.
- Limitations – no control group, bias, no longer-term follow-up.

Ramoser, G., Guoth-Gumberger, M., Baumgartner-Sigl, S., Zoeggeler, T., Scholl-Burgi, S., Karall, D. Frenotomy for tongue-tie (frenulum linguae breve) showed improved symptoms in the short- and long-term follow-up. *Acta Paediatrica* 10 April 2019 https://www.ncbi.nim.nih.gov/pubmed/30968969
- Retrospective study of 329 patients (295 infants and 34 children).
- Evaluation of symptoms, short-term and long-term outcomes.
- 60% of the infants (mean age 6 weeks) showed inadequate breastfeeding – sore nipples, poor weight gain, dribbling milk, reduced milk supply, inadequate latch during bottle-feeding and mastitis.
- In the 34 children predominant symptoms were articulation disorders, misaligned teeth, problems swallowing food.
- 141 provided short-term feedback: 86% reported improvement, 13% reported no change.
- 164 provided long term feedback: 82% reported improvement, 16% unchanged.
- One infant refused to feed for two hours post-procedure; one had a fever for one day.

Edmunds, J., Miles, S., Fulbrook, P. (2011) Tongue-tie and breastfeeding: A review of the literature. *Breastfeeding Review* 2011:19(1):19-26.
- Looked at 25 papers and concluded that 'frenotomy offered the best chance of improved and continued breastfeeding'.

Finnigan, V., Long, T. The effectiveness of frenulotomy on infant feeding outcomes: a systematic review. *Evidence Based Midwifery* June 2013
- Looked at 5 RCTs and 9 case studies and concluded that 'frenotomy offers long term improvements in over 50% of cases.'

Ito, Y. (2014) Does frenotomy improve breast-feeding difficulties in infants with ankyloglossia? *Pediatrics International*, 56: 497-505.
- Concluded that there is an 'overall moderate quality of evidence for the effectiveness of frenotomy for the treatment of breastfeeding difficulties'.

Acknowledgements

Writing a book, like being an IBCLC and tongue-tie practitioner, can be a lonely occupation. I would like to thank all of the parents who contributed to this book, both directly with accounts of your experiences and photographs, and indirectly through providing me with the opportunity to support you and learn from your journeys. I would also like to thank the Association of Breastfeeding Mothers for the opportunity to train and volunteer with them as a breastfeeding counsellor, which set me on this path.

Thanks also need to go to Mervyn Griffiths and Carolyn Westcott who trained me in tongue-tie division and supported me in the early years and without whom the challenges families with tongue-tied babies currently face would be much greater. Additional thanks to Anna Le Grange, Mags Kirk and Moraig Goodwin for the sections they contributed to this book.

Special thanks must go to my husband Jon and children Zara and Patrick for putting up with the disturbance my profession creates in our daily lives.

Finally, thank you to Pinter & Martin for having faith in me and giving me the encouragement to write this book.

References

Introduction

Messner, A. & Lalakea, M. (2000). Ankyloglossia: controversies in management. *International Journal of Pediatric Otorhinolaryngology*, Aug 31;54(2-3):123-31.

Callum, I.M. (1959). An Old Wives Tale. *British Medical Journal*, 2:498.

Hazelbaker, A. (2010). *Tongue-tie: Morphogenesis, Impact, Assessment and Treatment*. Ohio: Aidan and Eva Press.

Hogan, M., Westcott, C., & Griffiths, D.M. (2005). A randomised, controlled trial of division of tongue-tie in infants with feeding problems. *Journal of Paediatrics and Child Health*, 41(5-6):246-50.

IBLCE. (2019). *Prepare for IBCLC Certification*. Retrieved from International Board of Lactation Consultant Examiners: https://iblce.org/step-1-prepare-for-ibclc-certification/

Newman, J. (1997). *Breastfeeding and Guilt*. Retrieved from Canadian Breastfeeding Foundation: https://www.canadianbreastfeedingfoundation.org/basics/guilt.shtml

NICE. (2005). *Division of ankyloglossia (tongue-tie) for breastfeeding*. Retrieved from National Institute for Health and Care Excellence: https://www.nice.org.uk/guidance/ipg149

NICE. (2014). *Maternal and Child Nutrition Public Health Guideline (PH11)*. Retrieved from National Institute for Health and Care Excellence: https://www.nice.org.uk/guidance/ph11

NMC. (2004). *Standards of proficiency for specialist community public health nurses*. Retrieved from Nursing and Midwifery Council: https://www.nmc.org.uk/globalassets/sitedocuments/standards/nmc-standards-of-proficiency-for-specialist-community-public-health-nurses.pdf

NMC. (2009). *Standards for Pre-registration Midwifery Education*. Retrieved from Nursing and Midwifery Council: https://www.nmc.org.uk/globalassets/sitedocuments/standards/nmc-standards-for-preregistration-midwifery-education.pdf

UNICEF BFI. (1992). *History of Baby Friendly*. Retrieved from UNICEF UK The Baby Friendly Initiative: https://www.unicef.org.uk/babyfriendly/about/history/

WHO. (2003). *Global Strategy on Infant and Young Child Nutrition*. Retrieved from World Health Organisation: https://www.who.int/nutrition/publications/infantfeeding/9241562218/en/

Chapter 1: What is a tongue-tie?

Amitai et al, (2019) Pre-conceptional folic acid supplementation: A possible cause for the increasing rates of ankyloglossia https://www.sciencedirect.com/science/article/pii/S0306987719311259?fbclid=IwAR3Mocm-Kd6L5vMuFJx1z5_EN08I3QB0Ce34A0HOhSe89RffWrkgc96IUJU

Cullum (1959) An Old Wives Tale. *BMJ* 19 Sept 1959, p 497

Elad et al, (2014) Biomechanics of milk extraction during breast-feeding http://www.pnas.org/content/111/14/5230

Geddes et al, (2008) Frenulotomy for breastfeeding infants with ankyloglossia: effect on milk removal and sucking mechanism as imaged by ultrasound https://pubmed.ncbi.nlm.nih.gov/18573859/

Haham et al, (2014) Prevalence of Breastfeeding Difficulties in Newborns with a Lingual Frenulum: A Prospective Cohort Series https://www.researchgate.net/publication/265859110_Prevalence_of_Breastfeeding_Difficulties_in_Newborns_with_a_Lingual_Frenulum_A_Prospective_Cohort_Series

Hogan, M., Westcott, C., Griffiths, M. (2005) A randomised, controlled trial of division of tongue-tie in infants with feeding problems. *Journal of Paediatrics and Child Health*; 2005 https://www.ncbi.nlm.nih.gov/pubmed/15953322

Ingram et al, (2015) The development of a tongue assessment tool to assist with tongue-tie identification. https://fn.bmj.com/content/100/4/F344

Lin, S. Is tongue-tied genetic? Here is the Truth https://www.drstevenlin.com/tongue-tied-genetic/ (accessed 26/10/2020)

Martinelli et al, (2014) Histological Characteristics of Altered Human Lingual Frenulum http://savvysciencepublisher.com/downloads/ijpchv2n1a2/

Maya-Enero S, Perez_Perez M, Ruiz-Guzman L, et al (2020) Prevalence of neonatal ankyloglossia in a tertiary care hospital in Spain: a transversal cross-sectional study. European Journal of Pediatrics 2021 Mar;180(3):751-757. doi: 10.1007/s00431-020-03781-7.

Mills et al, (2019) What is a tongue tie? Defining the anatomy of the in-situ lingual frenulum https://onlinelibrary.wiley.com/doi/full/10.1002/ca.23343

Mills et al, (2019) Defining the anatomy of the neonatal lingual frenulum https://onlinelibrary.wiley.com/doi/full/10.1002/ca.23410

Perez-Aguirre B, et al (2018) Oral findings and its association with prenatal and perinatal factors in newborns. https://www.ncbi.nlm.nih.gov/pmc/articles/PMC6172521/

Todd, D., Hogan, M. (2015) Tongue-tie in the newborn: early diagnosis and division prevents poor breastfeeding outcomes. https://www.ncbi.nlm.nih.gov/pubmed/25906492

WHO (2001) The World Health Organization's Infant Feeding Recommendation https://www.who.int/nutrition/topics/infantfeeding_recommendation/en/

Chapter 2: The impact of tongue-tie on infant feeding

Brown, A., Jones, W. (2019) *A Guide to Supporting Breastfeeding for the Medical Profession*.

Brown, A., Jordan, S. (2012) Impact of birth complications on breastfeeding duration: an internet survey. *JAN* Volume 69, Issue 4 Pages: 745-983

Darmangeat, V. (2011) The Frequency and Resolution of Nipple Pain When Latch is Improved in a Private Practice. *Clinical Lactation* Vol 2, Issue 3.

Dezio, M. et al (2015) Tongue-tie, from embryology to treatment: a literature review. *Journal of Pediatric and Neonatal Individualized Medicine* 2015:4(1)

Elad, D. et al (2014) Biomechanics of milk extraction during breast-feeding http://www.pnas.org/content/111/14/5230

Geddes, D. et al (2008) Frenulotomy for breastfeeding infants with ankyloglossia: effect on milk removal and sucking mechanism as imaged by ultrasound https://pubmed.ncbi.nlm.nih.gov/18573859/

Genna, C.W., Saperstein, Y., Siegel, S.A., et al (2021) Quantitive imaging of tongue kinematics during infant feeding and adult swallowing reveals highly conserved patterns. *Physiological Reports*. vol 9 issue 3

Hayden, E. (2000) *Osteopathy for Children*

James, S. (2013) Human pain and genetics: some basics. *British Journal of Pain* 25 Sept 2013 https://doi.org/10.1177/2049463713506408

Kent, J.C. et al (2015) Nipple Pain in Breastfeeding Mothers: Incidence, Causes and Treatments. *Int J Environ Res Public Health* 2015 Sep 29;12(10):122247-63 https://pubmed.ncbi.nlm.nih.gov/26426034/

Lucas, R. (2019) Promoting self-management of breast and nipple pain in breastfeeding women: Protocol of a pilot randomized controlled trial. *Research in Nursing and Health* March 2019 DOI: 10.1002/nur.21938

Means-Christensen, A.J. (2008) Relationships among pain, anxiety, and depression in primary care. *Depress Anxiety* 2008;25(7):593-600 https://pubmed.ncbi.nlm.nih.gov/17932958/

Odent, M. (2013) Synthetic oxytocin and breastfeeding: Reasons for testing an hypothesis. *Medical Hypotheses* 81 (2013) 889-891

Sergueef, N. (2007) *Cranial Osteopathy for Infants, Children and Adolescents: A Practical Handbook*

Watson Genna, C. (2017) *Supporting Sucking Skills in Breastfeeding Infants*. 3rd Edition, 2017.

Chapter 3: Assessment and diagnosis of tongue-tie

Amir, L. et al (2006) Reliability of the Hazelbaker Assessment Tool for Lingual Frenulum Function. *International Breastfeeding Journal*,1,3.

Bergman, N. (2013) Neonatal stomach volume and physiology suggest feeding at 1-h intervals. *Acta Paediatrica* 10 May 2013

Coryllos, E., Watson Genna, C., Salloum, A.C. (2004) Newsletter of the American Academy of Pediatrics – Summer 2004

Ferres-Amat, E., Pastor-Vera, T., et al (2016) Multidisciplinary management of ankyloglossia in childhood. Treatment of 101 cases. A protocol. *Med Oral Patol Oral Cir Bucal*. 2016 Jan 1;21(1):e39-47. doi: 10.4317/medoral.20736. PMID: 26595832; PMCID: PMC4765751.

Griffiths, D.M. (2004) Do tongue ties affect breastfeeding? *Journal of Human Lactation*. 2004;20:411

Hester, S.N. et al (2012) Is the Macronutrient Intake of Formula-Fed Infants Greater Than Breast-Fed Infants in Early Infancy? *Journal of Nutrition and Metabolism* 2012 Article ID 891201

Ingram, J., Johnson, D., Copeland, M., et al (2015) The development of a tongue assessment tool to assist with tongue-tie identification. *Archives of Disease in Childhood – Fetal and Neonatal Edition* 2015;**100:**F344-F349.

Ingram, J., Copeland, M., Johnson, D. et al (2019) The development and evaluation of a picture tongue assessment tool for tongue-tie in breastfed babies (TABBY). *Int Breastfeed J* **14,** 31 (2019).

Jensen, D. (1994) LATCH: A Breastfeeding Charting System and Documentation Tool. *Journal of Obstetric, and Neonatal Nursing*. Jan 1994.

Lopes de Castro Martinelli, et al (2016) Validity and reliability of the neonatal tongue screening test. *Revista CEFAC*, 18(6), 1323-1331.

Mohrbacher, N. (2011) The Magic Number and Long-term Milk Production. *Clinical Lactation*, 2011, Vol. 2-1, 15-18

NHS Guidelines on Infant Formula Preparation www.nhs.uk/conditions/pregnancy-and-baby/making-up-infant-formula/ (accessed 28/10/20)

Srinivasan, A., Dobrich, C. et al (2006) Ankyloglossia in Breastfeeding Infants: The Effect of Frenotomy on Maternal Nipple Pain and Latch. *Breastfeeding Medicine* Vol 1, No 4.

Chapter 4: Treatment of tongue-tie

Brookes, A., Bowley, D.M. (2014) Tongue-tie: The evidence for frenotomy. *Early Human Development*. Volume 90, Issue 11, November 2014, Pages 765-768

Devishree et al (2012) Frenectomy: A Review with the Reports of Surgical Techniques. *Journal of Clinical and Diagnostic Research*. 2012 Nov; 6(9): 1587–1592

Griffiths, D.M. (2004) Do Tongue Ties Affect Breastfeeding? *Journal of Human Lactation*. Nov 2004. https://journals.sagepub.com/doi/abs/10.1177/0890334404266976

Hale, M. et al (2019) Complications following frenotomy for ankyloglossia: A 24-month prospective New Zealand Paediatric Surveillance Unit study. *Journal of Paediatrics and Child Health* Volume 56, Issue 4. https://onlinelibrary.wiley.com/doi/abs/10.1111/jpc.14682

Hazelbaker, A. (2010) *Tongue-tie: Morphogenesis, Impact, Assessment and Treatment*

Hogan, M., Westcott, C., Griffiths, M. (2005) A randomised, controlled trial of division of tongue-tie in infants with feeding problems. *Journal of Paediatrics and Child Health*; 2005 https://www.ncbi.nlm.nih.gov/pubmed/15953322

Illing, S. et al (2019) The value of frenotomy for ankyloglossia from a parental perspective. *The New Zealand Medical Journal*. Vol 132 No 1500: 16 August 2019

Mills et al (2019) What is a tongue tie? Defining the anatomy of the in-situ lingual frenulum https://onlinelibrary.wiley.com/doi/full/10.1002/ca.23343

Mills et al (2019) Defining the anatomy of the neonatal lingual frenulum https://onlinelibrary.wiley.com/doi/full/10.1002/ca.23410

Mills et al (2020) Understanding the Lingual Frenulum: Histological Structure, Tissue Composition, and Implications for Tongue Tie Surgery. *International Journal of Otolaryngology* Volume 2020 https://www.hindawi.com/journals/ijoto/2020/1820978/

Moore, E.R. et al (2012) Early skin-to-skin contact for mothers and their healthy newborn infants. *Cochrane Database of Systematic Reviews.*

NICE (2005) Division of ankyloglossia (tongue-tie) for breastfeeding. Interventional procedures guidance [IPG149] Published date: 14 December 2005

Opara, P.I., Gabriel-Job, N. & Opara, K.O. Neonates presenting with severe complications of frenotomy: a case series. *J Med Case Reports* **6,** 77 (2012). https://doi.org/10.1186/1752-1947-6-77

O'Shea, J.E. et al (2017) Frenotomy for tongue-tie in newborn infants. *Cochrane Database of Systematic Reviews.*

Papathanasiou, E. et al (2017) Current and Emerging Treatments for Postsurgical Cleft Lip Scarring: Effectiveness and Mechanisms. *Journal of Dental Research.* June 26, 2017

Shah, P.S. et al (2012) Breastfeeding or breast milk for procedural pain in neonates (Review). *Cochrane Database of Systematic Reviews*

Tasci, B., Kuzlu Ayyildiz, T. The Calming Effect of Maternal Breast Milk Odor on Term Infant: A Randomized Controlled Trial. *Breastfeed Med.* 2020 Nov;15(11):724-730. doi: 10.1089/bfm.2020.0116. Epub 2020 Oct 29. PMID: 33121256. https://pubmed.ncbi.nlm.nih.gov/33121256/https://www.liebertpub.com/doi/10.1089/bfm.2020.01...

The Australian Dental Association (2020) Ankyloglossia and Oral Frena Consensus Statement. https://www.ada.org.au/Dental-Professionals/Publications/Ankyloglossia-Statement/Ankyloglossia-and-Oral-Frena-Consensus-Statement_J.aspx

Chapter 5: Strategies to help a tongue-tied baby feed before and after division

Morton et al (2009) https://www.nature.com/articles/jp200987

Chapter 6: Myths and controversies

Dezio, M. et al (2015) Tongue-tie, from embryology to treatment: a literature review. *Journal of ''Pediatric and Neonatal Individualized Medicine* 2015;4(1):e040101

Baxter, R. et al (2020) Functional Improvements of Speech, Feeding, and Sleep After Lingual Frenectomy Tongue-Tie Release: A Prospective Cohort Study. *Clin Pediatr* (Phila) 2020 Sep;59(9-10):885-892.

Choi Yun-Seok, Lim Jin-Soo, Han Ki-Taik, et al (2011) Ankyloglossia Correction: Z-Plasty Combined With Genioglossus Myotomy. *The Journal of Cranial Surgery.* Vol 22, No 6, Nov 2011.

D'Onofiro, L. (2019) Oral dysfunction as a cause of malocclusion. *Orthodontics and Craniofacial Research.* 2019;22(Suppl. 1):43–48.

Ito, Y. et al (2015) Effectiveness of tongue-tie division for speech disorder in children. *Pediatrics International* 2015 Apr;57(2):222-6

Jang S-J. et al (2011) Relationship between the lingual frenulum and craniofacial morphology in adults. *Am J Orthod Dentofacial Orthop* 2011 Apr:139 (4 Suppl); e361-7

Johnson, P. (2006) Tongue-tie – exploding the myths. *Infant* vol 2, issue 3, 2006. https://www.infantjournal.co.uk/pdf/inf_009.pdf

Kotlow, L. (2015) TOTS–Tethered Oral Tissues The Assessment and Diagnosis of the Tongue and Upper Lip Ties

Mills, N., Lydon, A-M., Davies-Payne, D., et al (2020) Imaging the breastfeeding swallow: Pilot study utilizing real-time MRI. *Laryngoscope Investigative Otolaryngology.* Vol 5 Issue 3

Mohan, R., Soni, P.K., Krishna, M.K., Gundappa, M. (2014) Proposed classification of medial maxillary labial frenum based on morphology. *Dent Hypotheses* 2014;5:16-20.

Nakhash, R. et al (2019) Upper Lip Tie and Breastfeeding: A Systematic Review. *Breastfeeding Medicine* 2019 Mar;14(2):83-87

Townsend, J.A., Brannon, R.B., Cheramie, T., Hagan, J. (2013) Prevalence and variations of the median maxillary labial frenum in children, adolescents, and adults in a diverse population. *General Dentistry* March/April 2013

Salt, H. et al (2020) Speech production in young children with tongue-tie. *International Journal of Pediatric Otorhinolaryngology* Volume 134, July 2020, 110035

Vaz, A.C., Bai, P.M. (2015) Lingual frenulum and malocclusion: An overlooked tissue or a minor issue. *Indian Journal of Dental Research* Vol 26, Issue 5, p488-492

Index

adrenaline 88
After-Care Advice Sheet 74
air, baby taking in (aerophagia) 31, 35, 53, 54
Amir, L. 65
Amitai, Y. 22
Ankyloglossia and Oral Frena Consensus Statement (Australian Dental Association) 103
anterior tongue-ties 17, 24, 33, 67–9
anxiety 46–9, 143
apoptosis 21, 22
arched palate 37, 38, 122
assessment for tongue-tie 7–8, 18–20, 23–4, 55–69, 78–9
Assessment Tool for Lingual Frenulum Function 18–19
assessment tools 18–19, 64–6
Association of Breastfeeding Mothers 10, 124, 125
Association of Tongue-tie Practitioners (ATP) 74, 87–8
asymmetry of face or head 41

Bai, P.M. 136
Baldwin, Nicholas 89
Barbour Andrews, Vicky 62
base of skull 44, 45
base of tongue, tension in 68
Baxter, Richard 135
Bergman, Nils J. 58
birth, checks at 7–8
birth interventions 40–1, 43, 50, 112
bleeding (post-division) 82, 85–9
bleeding disorders 87–8, 103
bleeding nipples 39
blisters on lips 28
blocked ducts 29
blood clotting 86–7
body workers 54, 121, 125
bottle-feeding *see also* formula feeding
    impact of tongue-tie on 32–3
    and lack of acknowledgement of tongue-tie as an issue 12
    overfeeding 50–1, 53, 118–19
    paced bottle-feeding 54, 119, 122
    positioning 61
    strategies to help child feed 122
Bowley, D.M. 78
Brazil 16, 73

breast abscesses 29–30
breast anatomy 23–4
breast compression 120–1
breast implants 25, 52
breast pain 29 *see also* nipple pain
breast pumps 40, 115–16
breast refusal 95–6
breast shaping technique 40, 109–10
breast storage capacity 60
breast surgery 51–2
breastfeeding
    antibodies 90
    and birth complications 40–1
    creation of negative pressure 21
    education 61
    feeding assessment 8, 54, 59–64, 106
    impact of tongue-tie on 27–54
    as learned skill 61, 123
    maternal anatomy 23–4
    milk supply 49–53
    as pain relief immediately after division 92–4
    post-division 74, 98
    rates of (UK) 36
    role of the tongue in 20–1
    specialist breastfeeding support 125–6
    strategies to help child feed 105–26
    sub-optimal breastfeeding management 49–51
    support for 10, 13, 99–100, 106, 123–5
    and tongue extension 20
    and tongue lift 20
    trauma and grief 142
    underinvestment in 10
Breastfeeding Assessment Tools 124
Breastfeeding Network 10, 125
Bristol Tongue Assessment Tool 65–6, 67
British Medical Journal 12, 23
Brodie director 25, 71
Brookes, A. 78
Brown, Amy 40–1, 142
bubble palate 37, 38
buccal tie 131–2

Callum, I.M. 12, 23
Cameron, Angus 131
causes of tongue-tie 21–2, 68
CHINS (latching principles) 106–7

chiropractors 41, 79, 82, 121
choking 31, 65
cleft palate 22, 49, 103, 104
clicking sound 28, 35, 54, 64
'cobble stone' lip blisters 28
Cochrane systematic reviews 92, 95, 97
colic 53–4
collagen 17, 73, 75
comfort sucking 119
'coming in,' milk 50
commonness of tongue-tie 23–6
compensations, baby making 28, 114, 129
compensations, mother making 62
coordination issues 67
cord round the neck 40, 45–6
cortisol 93
Coryllos, Betty 24
cow's milk protein allergy 53
cranial osteopathy 42, 79
cranial sacral therapists 41, 121
crying 19–20, 92, 94
C-section births 40–1, 43–4, 87
cup feeding 120
cupping of the tongue 27–8, 35, 64, 65
cutting a tongue-tie see divisions
cysts 96

Darmangeat, Veronique 35
dental issues 33, 68, 130, 131, 136–7
dentistry 128
depression 46–9
Devishree, S.K.G. 95
Dezio, M. 33, 136
diabetes 51–2
diagnosis of tongue-tie 24, 34–5, 55–69
diamond-shaped wound 82, 83
disruptive wound massage (DWM) 74–8
divisions
    bleeding 82, 85–9
    breastfeeding as pain relief 93–4
    complications from 86
    contraindications to 103–4
    efficacy of 97–100
    exercises for after 74
    impact on bottle-feeding 33
    incomplete divides 82–3
    infection 89–92
    of lip ties 129–31
    making the decision to 56
    not always the answer 25–6, 65, 103–4
    in older children/adults 68–9, 70, 80,

136, 137
    pain 80, 92–5
    professional assessment 55
    re-divisions 73, 76, 78–84
    risk of damage 96
    statistics on need for 24–5
    stories with less successful outcomes 102–3
    success stories 100–2
    types of procedures 70–1
    unnecessary 26
    when treatment doesn't improve things 138–43
    wound healing 18, 72, 74–81, 88, 89–92, 136
    Z-plasty 68–9
Dobrich, Carole 65
doctors see healthcare professionals
D'Onofrio, Linda 132
donor milk 117
Down's syndrome 104
drainage of the breast, effective/ineffective 29–30, 50
dribbling milk during a feed 28
dummies/pacifiers 94
dynamic structure, lingual frenulum as 17–18

efficient transfer of milk 29–30, 49, 106
Elad, David 20–1, 45
elasticity of frenulum 65
elastin 73
electro cautery 70–1, 89
engorgement 29
epidurals 40
Equality Act 2010 36
exaggerated latch (flipple/nipple flick) 108–9
expressing 51, 114–20

facial massage 80
families, support for 123–5
families, tongue-tie running in 21 see also genetic factors; siblings
fast flowing milk 30–1, 35
feeding assessment 8, 54, 59–64, 106
Ferres-Amat, E 68
fibrousness of tongue-ties 73
finger-feeding 95, 119, 120
finger-sucking games 74
'fire hose' feeding 30
flanged lips 129
flat head syndrome (plagiocephaly) 45

flat/inverted nipples 39–40
flipple/nipple flick 108–9
floppy larynx (laryngomalacia) 49, 104
flow regulation 30–1, 35, 53, 54, 65
folic acid 21–2
forceps/ventouse births 40–1, 43, 112
forces of labour 41–6
formula feeding *see also* bottle-feeding
    frequency of feeds 59–60
    and lack of acknowledgement of
        tongue-tie as an issue 12
    post-division 98
    risk of infection 90
    safe preparation of 90
    top-ups 49–50, 117–18
frenectomy 70–1
Frenotomy Decision Tool for
    Breastfeeding Dyads 65
frenulotomy/frenotomy 70, 71–2
frenulum *see* labial frenulum; lingual
    frenulum
frequency of feeds 29, 35, 50–1, 58–9,
    73–4

gag reflex 122
galactagogues 117
gas/wind 30, 31, 35
Geddes, D. 20, 29
general anaesthetic 70
genetic factors 21, 23, 38
genioglossus muscle 68, 82, 83, 97, 136
Goodwin, Moraig 42–6
Griffiths, Mervyn 13, 69, 82, 92
'growing back' a tongue-tie 72–3
gulping 31, 64
gut bacteria 87

Haham, Alon 24
Hale, M. 86
hand expressing 115–16
'happy spitters' 53
Hayden, E. 42, 43, 44
Hazelbaker, Alison 11, 17, 18–19, 21, 65,
    72, 130
Hazelbaker Tool for Lingual Frenulum
    Function (HATLFF) 18, 25, 65
head, baby's, strain/tension of birth on
    41–6
head shape 41
healing by secondary intention 75–6
healthcare professionals
    assessment for tongue-tie 56
    skill in identifying tongue-tie 8–9

training in infant feeding 10–12
training in tongue-tie 57
heart/lung conditions 49, 104
Hearts Milk Bank 117
heart-shaped tongue 34, 62
Heinig, M.J. 59
Hester, S.N. 59
high arched palate 37, 38, 122
Hill, P.D. 116
Hogan, Monica 8, 9, 18, 24, 92
hormonal disorders 51–2
how many babies have tongue tie 23–6
'hugging' of the breast with tongue 27–8
    see also cupping of the tongue
Human Milk for Human Babies 118
humping of tongue 28
hyoid bone 33, 45–6
hypoglossal nerve 79
hypoplasia of the breasts 25, 52–3

IBCLCs (International Board Certified
    Lactation Consultants)
    assessment for tongue-tie 9, 55–6
    breastfeeding support 13, 123–5
    as part of multidisciplinary approach
        54
    training in infant feeding 11, 56
Illing, S. 98
incidence rates 23–6
ineffective draining of the breast 29–30
inefficient feeding 29–30, 35
infant feeding, impact of tongue-tie on
    27–54
infant paracetamol 94
infection 77, 89–92
inflammation 75, 76
Ingram, Jenny 23, 65, 66
insufficient glandular tissue 25, 52–3
inverted/flat nipples 39–40

James, Sabu 48
Jang, S-J. 136
jaundice 105–6
jaw anatomy 24, 33, 38, 104
jaw assessment 44
jaw tension 37, 67, 99, 121
Jenson, Deborah 57–8
Johnson, Paul 136–7
Jordan, S. 40–1

Kangaroo care 95
Kent, J.C. 35
Kirk, Mags 132
Klebsiella oxytoca 89–90

Kotlow, Larry 128

La Leche League 10, 124, 125
labial frenulum 127–8
lactation aids 119–20
laid-back feeding positions 54, 107–8
Lalakea, M. 13
laryngomalacia (floppy larynx) 49, 104
laser divisions 70–1, 89, 95, 96
latch
      assessing 64
      babies who will not 112–14
      CHINS (latching principles) 106–7
      effective 106–7, 110–11
      feeding assessment 57–8
      flat/inverted nipples 39–40
      impact of tongue-tie on 27, 28–9,
            34, 35–6
      lip position 128–9
      role of the tongue in 20–1
      and the Temporo-Mandibular Joint
            44
LATCH (assessment tool) 57–8
latch assist devices 40
latching in motion 113
lateralisation of the tongue 19, 33, 65,
      74, 133
Le Grange, Anna 47
length of feeds 29 see also frequency of
      feeds
'let down' reflex 30, 54, 112
'letter box' mouth 20
Lin, Steven 22
lingual frenulum
      anatomy of 15–18, 23, 72, 92
      anterior versus posterior tongue ties
            67–9
      assessing 64–7
      causes of tongue=tie 21–2
      divisions - types 70–1
lingual nerve damage 82, 96–7
Linthicum-Watson, Amy 63
lip blisters 28
lip tie 66, 127–31
lipstick-shaped nipples 28, 62
liver disease 87, 103
local anaesthetic 70, 92, 94
Lopez de Castro Martinelli, R. 16, 65
low muscle tone 49, 67, 104, 126
Lucas, Ruth 48

Marasco, Lisa 117
Marcheson, Irene 16

Martinelli, R.L.C 16, 65
massage
      facial/jaw 80–1
      of the wound 74–8
mastitis 29, 49
maternal anxiety 46–9, 143
Maya-Enero, S. 24–5
Means-Christensen, A.J. 46
Messner, A 13, 148
microbiome 87
midwives see healthcare professionals
milk ejection reflex 30, 41, 54
milk supply 30, 49–53, 60, 114–15
Mills, Nikki 17–18, 21, 68, 73, 83, 92,
      96, 129
mindfulness 47
misshapen nipples 24, 28–9, 37, 62
Mohan, R. 127
Mohrbacher, N. 60
Morton, J. 116
Moss, William 12–13
mother, support for 122–5
mouth opening ability 19, 44–5
MTHFR gene mutation 21–2
multidisciplinary assessment 54, 126
Murnane, Dermot 89
muscle fatigue 80, 94–5
muscular tension 68, 74, 78, 80
myotomy 136

Nakhash, R. 130
nappies 111
nasogastric tubes 32, 119
NCT 124
neck strain 20, 41, 74, 79
negative pressure 21, 27, 29
Neonatal Infant Pain Score 93
Neonatal Tongue Screening Test 65–6
neuromuscular conditions 103, 104
Newborn and Infant Physical
      Examination (NIPE) 7–8
Newman, Jack 15–16, 78, 120
NHS services 78
NICE (The National Institute for Health
      and Care Excellence)
      Guidance on Division of Ankyloglossia
            for Breastfeeding 9, 13, 89, 97
      Guidance on Maternal and Child
            Nutrition 9
nipple blanching 28–9, 37–8
nipple flattening 28
nipple mis-shaping 24, 28–9, 37, 62

nipple pain
    feeding assessment 61–2
    flat/inverted nipples 39–40
    impact of tongue-tie on 20, 28–9, 34, 35–6
    maternal anxiety 46–9
    as measure of efficacy of division 97–8
    palate shape 37, 38
    thrush 36–7
    vasospasm 37–8
nipple shields 39–40, 113–14
NMC (Nursing and Midwifery Council) 10
NPEU, Oxford University 99–100
nursing pillows 107

obesity 60
Odent, Michel 41
oesophageal sphincter (stomach valve) 53
one-sided strain patterns 45
Opara, P.I. 86
oral aversion 71, 77
oral mucosa 16–17
O'Shea, J.E. 97
osteopathy 41, 42, 44–6, 54, 79, 82, 99, 121
over-diagnosis of tongue-tie 56
overfeeding 53, 60, 118
over-granulation of wound 91–2
oversupply 54
oxytocin 41, 117
paced bottle-feeding 54, 119, 122

pacifiers/dummies 94
pain (maternal) 46–9 see also breast pain; nipple pain
pain, of a division 80, 92–5
pain relief medication
    for a division 62, 94
    in labour (effects on baby) 40–1
palate shape 37, 38, 49
Papathanasiou, E. 76
paracetamol 94
Perez-Aguire, B. 22
peristaltic (wave) motion 21, 27, 32, 35, 39, 65
Pierre Robin Sequence 103, 104
pitocin/syntocinon 40
plagiocephaly (flat head syndrome) 45
polycystic ovary syndrome (PCOS) 51–2
positioning (during birth) 42–3
positioning and attachment (feeding) 35,

36, 40, 61, 62, 106–8
posterior tongue ties 17, 18, 24, 33, 57, 67–9
post-natal depression 46–7
power pumping 116
progesterone 50
prolactin 112, 115
Puckering, Holly 129
pumping milk 40, 115–16 see also expressing

race 49
ranula 96
rapid labour 43
rates of tongue-tie 23–6
Raynaud's phenomenon 38
rebirthing 112–13
recessed lower jaw 24
recurrence of tongue tie 17, 72–4, 136
referral pathways 56
reflux symptoms 31, 32, 35, 53–4, 95
relaxation techniques 47–8
Rosen von Rosenstein, Nils 12

salivary glands 83, 96
Salt, H. 135
scarring 17, 72, 73, 76, 81, 83
scepticism about tongue-tie 12, 13–14, 61
scissors, using to divide a tie 70, 71, 92
seal at the breast 28, 31, 35, 54, 64 see also vacuum creation
seal on a bottle teat 122
sensory processing issues 125–6
sepsis 89
Sergueef, N. 44, 45, 46
Shah, P.S. 92–3
shallow latch 28–9, 36, 39
short, very frequent feeding 29
siblings 98, 142–3
side-lying feeding positions 108
Siegel, Scott 31, 53
skin colour 49
skin-to-skin 95, 108, 112, 113
Slagter, Kirsten 53
sleep cycles 59
slipping back, tongue 28
slow labour 43
slow weight gain 30, 35, 49–51, 58
snapback of the tongue 28, 35, 65
solids, starting 33–4
specialist clinics 57
speech and language therapy 54
speech impairments 68, 132–6

spitting up/vomiting after feeds 30, 51, 53
Srinivasan, A. 65
Standards of Proficiency for Specialist Community Public Health Nurses (Health Visitors) 10
stitches (sutures) 71
stool output 111
strabismus scissors 71
strain and tension from birth 41–6, 68, 79, 81–2, 121
stress 47–8
sub-mandibular ducts, damage to 96
sub-mucosal tongue-ties 24, 68 *see also* posterior tongue ties
sub-optimal breastfeeding management 49–51
suck reflex 39
'suck to swallow' ratio 58
sucrose solution (for pain management) 93
suction devices 40
supplementary nursing systems 119–20
surgeons, referral to 54, 56, 83, 96
sutures 71
symptom list for tongue-tie 34–5 *see also* assessment for tongue-tie; diagnosis of tongue-tie
syntocinon/pitocin 41
syringe feeding 119
systematic reviews 92, 95, 97, 98

Tasci, B. 93
teats (bottles) 32–3, 90, 119, 122
teeth/dental issues 33, 68, 130, 131, 136–7
Temporo-Mandibular Joint (TMJ) 44 *see also* jaw anatomy
tension and strain from birth 41–6, 68, 79, 81–2, 121
thrush 36–7, 38
thyroid issues 51–2
tiring, baby finds feeding 29, 35, 58, 64, 80
Todd, David 24
tongue damage 96
tongue extension 19, 20, 27, 28, 34, 65, 108
tongue function assessment 64–7
tongue lift 19–20, 35, 65, 80
tongue poking 79–80
tongue resting posture 133
tongue stability 133
tongue tone 80, 98

tongue-poking games 74
tongue-thrust reflex 33–4
Tongue-tie and Breastfed Babies Assessment Tool 65–6, 67
tongue-tip position 33–4, 38, 65, 133
Townsend, J.A. 127
trauma 142–3
tremor in the tongue 29
tube feeding 119–20
tubular breasts 52
tummy time 79, 121–2
'type one/two/three' ties 69

ulceration 90–1
UNICEF
    Baby Friendly 9, 10–11, 13, 16, 56
    Breastfeeding Assessment Tools 59
    description of tongue tie 16
upright positions for feeding 54

vacuum creation 20, 29, 30, 35, 49
vasospasm 37–8
Vaz, A.C. 136
ventouse/forceps births 40–1, 43, 112
vitamin A 22
vitamin K 86–7, 103
vomiting after feeds 30, 51, 53

Watson Genna, Catherine 24, 28, 32, 68, 69, 129
wave (peristaltic) motion 21, 27, 32, 35, 39, 65
weight gain (baby) 30, 35, 49–51, 56, 58
West, Diana 117
Westcott, Carolyn 94
wet nappies 111
white coating on tongue 38, 66
white nipples *see* nipple blanching
WHO (World Health Organisation)
    Global Strategy on Infant and Young Child Nutrition 13
    Recommendation on Infant Feeding 10, 26
wind/gas 30, 31, 35
wound healing 18, 72, 74–81, 88, 89–92, 136
wound stretches 74–8

Yasmin, Effath 95

Zaghi, Soroush 69
Z-plasty 71, 135–6

*Available from Pinter & Martin
in the **Why it Matters** series*

1   *Why Your Baby's Sleep Matters* Sarah Ockwell-Smith

2   *Why Hypnobirthing Matters* Katrina Berry

3   *Why Doulas Matter* Maddie McMahon

4   *Why Postnatal Depression Matters* Mia Scotland

5   *Why Babywearing Matters* Rosie Knowles

6   *Why the Politics of Breastfeeding Matter* Gabrielle Palmer

7   *Why Breastfeeding Matters* Charlotte Young

8   *Why Starting Solids Matters* Amy Brown

9   *Why Human Rights in Childbirth Matter* Rebecca Schiller

10 *Why Mothers' Medication Matters* Wendy Jones

11 *Why Home Birth Matters* Natalie Meddings

12 *Why Caesarean Matters* Clare Goggin

13 *Why Mothering Matters* Maddie McMahon

14 *Why Induction Matters* Rachel Reed

15 *Why Birth Trauma Matters* Emma Svanberg

16 *Why Oxytocin Matters* Kerstin Uvnäs Moberg

17 *Why Breastfeeding Grief and Trauma Matter* Amy Brown

18 *Why Postnatal Recovery Matters* Sophie Messager

19 *Why Pregnancy and Postnatal Exercise Matter* Rehana Jawadwala

20 *Why Baby Loss Matters* Kay King

21 *Why Infant Reflux Matters* Carol Smyth

22 *Why Tongue-tie Matters* Sarah Oakley

23 *Why Formula Feeding Matters* Shel Banks

24 *Why Breech Birth Matters* Julia Fotherby

Series editor: Susan Last

pinterandmartin.com